P9-ASG-210

WHY SHOULD I EAT BETTER?

SIMPLE ANSWERS TO ALL YOUR NUTRITIONAL QUESTIONS

LISA MESSINGER

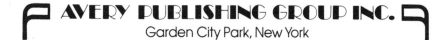
AVERY PUBLISHING GROUP INC.
Garden City Park, New York

Cover Design: Ann Vestal
Typesetting: Bonnie Freid
Printer: Paragon Press, Honesdale, PA

For Joel.

For, of course, all-important love. But also for what is often just slightly less important to the especially busy author: Doing the grocery shopping and laundry, taking in the dry cleaning, living in dust, moving into and out of whatever rooms are necessary, and being tremendously supportive and encouraging through it all.

Library of Congress Cataloging-in-Publication Data

Messinger, Lisa, 1962–
    Why should I eat better? : simple answers to all your
  nutritional questions / Lisa Messinger.
     p. cm.
  Includes bibliographical references and index.
  ISBN 0-89529-508-3
  1. Nutrition. I. Title.
RA784.M475 1993   92-33752
613.2—dc20   CIP

Printed in the United States of America

10 9 8 7 6 5 4 3 2

Contents

Part I   Why You Should Eat Better

Part II   How You Can Eat Better

Acknowledgments

Much thanks to Rudy Shur, president of Avery Publishing Group, for saying that he always wanted to publish a book like this, and to Arthur Vidro and Marie Caratozzolo, the sensitive and intelligent editors at Avery Publishing Group with whom I also worked. Thank you to my literary agents Theresa Cavanaugh and Jean Naggar, and to a great base newspaper, the *Antelope Valley Press*.

Preface

In a recent issue of *People* magazine on the "Picks & Pans Plus" page, next to such listings as "Dr. Ruth's Top 10 Favorite Romantic Movies" and "Tony Bennett's Top 10 Favorite Love Songs," was a list entitled "Top 10 Selling Diet Books."

The book list was just another piece of trivia stationed near "Top 10 Reasons People File for an Extension on Their Tax Returns." Unfortunately, many such books, which often rely on a special "new" diet angle or mysterious diet "secret," become fodder for trivia lists—or become virtually obsolete—almost as soon as they are published.

The popular comic strip character "Cathy," produced by Cathy Guisewite, is, like many people, a failed veteran of the diet wars. When it comes to food, this supposed prototype of today's modern, independent woman is also a confused shopper. A recent strip had her stationed in a supermarket cereal aisle having the following conversation with herself:

"Oat Flakes . . . Oatmeal Flakes . . . Oat Bran Flakes . . . Oat Bran Os . . . Oaties . . . Oat Squares . . . Crispy Oats . . . Honey Bunch of Oats . . . Honey Graham Ohs . . . Honey Nut Cheerios . . . Nut & Honey Crunch . . . Fruit 'N Bran Crunch . . . Crunchy Bran . . . Cracklin' Oat Bran . . . Common Sense Oat Bran . . . Super Bran . . . Raisin Bran . . . Bran Flakes . . . Fruitful Bran . . . All-Bran . . . 40+ Bran . . . 100% Bran . . . 100% Bran with Oat Bran . . . Bran Chex . . . Total

Raisin Bran ... Crispy Wheats 'N Raisins ... Shredded Wheat 'N Bran ... Bran Muesli ... Five Grain Muesli ... Muesli with Raisins, Peaches and Pecans ... One chocolate doughnut, please."

Cathy ends up in a doughnut shop. After surveying all those cereal choices—some of them undoubtedly healthful—she gives up in confusion over having so many choices and ends up eating what famed nutrition authority Jane Brody and others have named as one of the ten worst foods of all time. It's a food that's so detrimental to good nutrition that Brody says it's better not to eat breakfast at all than to eat a doughnut. Even if you are not in the doughnut shop of life, even if your library isn't the home of once-vogue diet books that now sport cobwebs, if you're a living, breathing consumer today, chances are you have some valid nutrition questions.

Never before has the country been so health and diet conscious. Food manufacturers are responding to that consciousness. "No cholesterol." "High fiber." "Oat bran." "No tropical oils." Packages all over market shelves—supermarket and health food store alike—have such labels.

But what does it all really mean? Out of the array of cooking oils available, which are the most healthful? Is fiber all it's cracked up to be, and, if so, what are its best sources? What is MSG? What does caffeine do once it's inside your body? Are the "fake fats" and new sweeteners we're hearing so much about good for your health? They're certainly popping up in more and more products.

At no time has it been more important to be an expert about such products. Study after study has shown that what we eat can affect not only how we feel, but possibly how long we live. Many of us have become "mini-experts." We know a lot about some things we had never even heard of until a few years ago: cholesterol, triglycerides, osteoporosis. *Why Should I Eat Better?* is designed to be a quick, concise guidebook to all the nutrition decisions we face every day. It gives answers to "Why should I eat better?" and "How can I eat better?" and looks at specific plans of action that can help us avoid cancer, heart disease, and other killers shown to have connections to diet.

As a health and nutrition columnist and investigative health reporter, I have broken many health and nutrition stories for my newspaper, the *Antelope Valley Press*.

Some of these stories, distributed worldwide through magazines, books, and the Los Angeles Times syndicate, might have played a part in making you a "mini-expert" on health and nutrition. However, I still saw the need to provide an accessible, easy-to-read, overall nutrition guide.

Similarly, Avery Publishing Group has had the opportunity to make nutrition and health news with many of its lauded health books. But, in these times of confusing health and nutrition claims, it also saw the need for a comprehensive, basic nutrition answer book. So, after I completed *The Tofu Book: The New American Cuisine* for Avery, Rudy Shur, Avery's managing editor, invited me to write this book.

I accepted. Being a food editor at a daily newspaper, as well as a reporter, I have access to the latest nutrition news. I am thrilled to share such news—possibly life-saving news—with you.

Introduction

There is $400 billion floating around out there trying to get you to eat processed food. (Processed food is the largest industry in the United States.) There were 470 million coupons trying to induce you to buy Nabisco's Teddy Grahams Breakfast Bears cereal when it was first introduced in 1989. There were 6,000 stores offering samples of the children's cereal, and for 17 weeks after Teddy Grahams was introduced, "Rockin' Bears" 30-second television commercials—one for mothers and one for children—aired in prime, day, after-school, and Saturday-morning time periods. Food advertising is a $3.6 billion annual industry in this country, and almost a third of the ads include some type of health claim.

When you're up against numbers like $400 billion, 470 million coupons, and 6,000 stores, just what kind of numbers would it take to get some real, unbiased, essential nutritional information? Believe it or not, that number is just one. You. Nutrition is an area where the slogan "looking out for number one" couldn't be more appropriate. Sometimes, all the conflicting information we hear about nutrition can get confusing. However, the key to caring for your health may be much simpler than you ever dreamed.

For example, the simple act of attempting to obtain more information could save or prolong your life. The University of Minnesota School of Public Health in Minneapolis reported that all it took was men going out and getting medical counseling on nutrition, smoking, or hypertension to boost their chances for a longer life. Those men had a 24 percent lower rate for heart attack, a 10.6 percent lower rate for coronary heart disease, and a 7.7 percent lower death rate overall than men who didn't get such counseling.

And speaking of the number one, and of simple acts, you might want to take the simple step of arming yourself with one carrot, just one carrot, a day.

That's because a study from the State University of New York at Buffalo compared the diets of 450 male lung cancer patients with the diets of over 900 healthy people. The men in the study whose beta-carotene intake was lowest were 80 percent more likely to have lung cancer than those with the highest. And just what was the difference between high and low carotene intakes? The equivalent of one carrot per day.

Of course, good nutrition and the prevention of cancer, heart disease, and other maladies involve a lot more than trying to eat a carrot a day. This book is all about trying to make the most of every day, and the rest of your life, by learning to make wise and life-lengthening food choices. If one carrot can make such a difference, a book packed with essential nutrition information should certainly have some impact.

And you deserve all the accurate information you can get. According to the Food Marketing Institute, as of 1991 the average family of four spent about $91 a week on food. Another survey shows that figure to be between 10 to 20 percent of the family of four's weekly salary. Another Food Marketing Institute survey of 750 adults found they spent an average of 56 minutes preparing dinner nightly. Over 40 percent of those questioned spent more than 45 minutes fixing the meal. With all that money and time invested in preparing meals, many people consciously try to put foods that are healthful into their shopping baskets. In fact, the Food Marketing Institute's survey showed that anxiety about dietary fat rose 17 percent in 1990 over 1989 levels. Almost two-thirds of shoppers said they wanted to improve their diets in all areas and were targeting their shopping to do so.

With today's emphasis on convenience and time-saving, why should you be wasting precious time and money on products that you think are healthful but whose health claims may merely be the product of an advertising copywriter's zealous imagination?

Do you think that food technologists—the people who develop new foods—and food advertisers basically try to present their foods to you honestly? I have studied hundreds of food labels and investigated many companies and have found honesty not always to be the case. But a recent annual meeting I covered of the country's largest group of food technologists (more than 25,000 members) hammered that point home to me even more.

I attended a lecture where a lawyer gave the group tips on how they could walk the fine line between puffery and out-and-out illegal deception in food product advertising. He was outlining how they could become expert at puffery.

Do you think a food product is introduced into the market simply because the company thinks it will be a hit with you and other food consumers? That same food technologists' meeting taught me differently. A food developer at the country's largest "salty snacks" company (as he repeatedly called it) described how one chip snack was almost not released, although it had tested very highly with consumer groups. The company, he said, was afraid the chips might be a little too spicy, so consumers might not eat (or buy) as much as they would of a less spicy chip. Eventually, consumers were brought in and told they were evaluating a thirty-minute travelogue. They were given the chips as snacks while they watched the film. The company was, in fact, testing the chips and heard enough crunching to decide to bring them to market, where they are currently a popular product.

This book tries to shed some light on the sometimes immense difference between popular products and those that use ingredients that are truly healthful. It might help you improve your shot at living a long and healthy life.

Right now, there seems to be a big roadblock on the boulevard leading to good nutritional health and possible longevity. That roadblock is confusion, which seems to be the current catchword in the press. "The nutritional awakening of the 1980s created a lot of confusion," read a large headline in the *Los Angeles Times* in January 1990.

The Associated Press reported: "Most Americans want nutritionally sound meals for themselves and their families but don't have a good enough understanding of nutrition to do so, according to a survey conducted by the Post Center for Nutrition and

Health. The survey asked 1,000 adults what questions they want answered about nutrition. More than half the responses showed a misunderstanding or lack of information, and 14 percent reflected a high level of confusion."

Another wire report on nutrition confusion concluded, "Despite their evident confusion and frustration about choosing the right foods for family health, 88 percent of the population persists in the quest for an ideal, balanced food plan."

I hope you're not confused at all by the seemingly conflicting nutrition information that bombards us every day. Perhaps you're just picking up this guidebook as a welcome addendum to your already extensive nutrition knowledge.

But who could blame you or anyone else if you did have some nutrition questions? In 1989, over 10,000 new grocery and household products were introduced—many with special health and nutritional claims. And what kind of advice are you often given to help you sort through it all? Well, *USA Today*, the country's biggest-circulation national newspaper, in a headline on a recent cover of its "Life" section, summed it up this way: "Top diet tack: Eat sensibly." In this day of high fiber, low cholesterol, no saturated fats, artificial this, and artificial that, what does that diet tack really mean? Unfortunately, much of the nutrition advice we hear is simply too general to make a real difference in our lives.

This book goes beyond the usual "eat sensibly" jargon. It looks at why you should eat better and how you can eat better, and briefly and simply delves into such topics as cholesterol, caffeine, MSG, vegetarianism, macrobiotics, artifical sweeteners, and the new "fake fats." It provides specific plans of dietary action that might prevent such killers as cancer and heart disease, as well as such problems as weight gain, osteoporosis, and food allergies.

In the *USA Today* article that told people to "eat sensibly," a Gallup poll of over 1,000 former dieters found only 117 of them successful. Their best advice: Cut out snacks and desserts and eat less.

This book takes a bold nutritional turn. It shows you how to *eat more* and not cut out healthful snacks and desserts. It helps you make sure all your food is packed with the most healthful ingredients available to ensure vitality, lifelong weight control, and longevity.

Part I

Why You Should Eat Better: What the Right Diet Can Prevent or Overcome

1

Diet and Your Health

Mary Xinh Nguyen should have a lot of strong memories. After all, the young Amerasian woman fled Vietnam in 1976; and in 1989, while still in her junior year at Boston University, she was named Revlon's Most Unforgettable Woman, winning $25,000 and a national appearance as a Revlon model.

Those are the makings of some strong memories. However, one of her strongest memories involves food. After boarding a bus in Vietnam and eventually making it to the United States by herself, Nguyen said, her foster family brought her to their home in St. Louis. She was very hungry, so the family tried to feed her some commercial spaghetti and brightly colored gelatin. She said, however, that the food was "really strange for someone from Asia. I didn't eat anything, because I thought they were trying to poison me."

Perhaps Nguyen, who later adapted to American food, doesn't realize how perceptive her first reactions had been. Although the enriched flours that make up most spaghetti products and the artificial colors, flavors, fillers, and sugars that go into many gelatins probably wouldn't have poisoned her that day, perhaps some inner voice was telling her that a lifetime of eating an array of these and other such foods could, in fact, play a part in poisoning her system.

Dr. Harry Demopoulis, a New York University Medical Center

pathologist and associate professor of pathology, has spent thirty years researching how people can avoid the fates of the 2,000 people whose autopsies he has performed. He thinks the "poisons" of the standard American diet show their true ravages in people by the time they are 35.

"The aorta is like a garden hose that runs along the spinal cavity," Demopoulis said of the artery that carries blood from the heart to the body's organs. "When you open it up, instead of finding a nice smooth lining, I've found lumps of ulcerated, bleeding pulps, like bloody scabs. Blood vessels are damaged, also. You see this in people because the American diet causes changes. Blood vessels in almost everyone over 35 are a mess."

It's too bad most of us can't participate in a few autopsies and see firsthand the damage a poor diet can do. And most of us never share Nguyen's perspective of entering the country with fresh eyes and being astounded at what seem to be dangerous food choices. Unfortunately, we're often pushed into such a diet virtually from birth.

But nothing dictates we have to follow such a diet mindlessly. Picking up a book like this shows that you care about your health and likely are aware of the possible relation between diet and certain diseases. Bravo. Read on, and reinforce your knowledge about (or be shocked by learning for the first time) just how many deaths and diseases might be avoided by manipulating our diets.

DEADLY NUMBERS

Unlike Demopoulis, Dr. Kenneth Kizer, M.P.H., doesn't preside over the autopsies of the 400 people he knows of who die each day. But he is just as concerned with what the insides of their tattered aortas and body organs look like.

Kizer, former director of the California Department of Health Services, estimates that during his tenure, about 400 Californians who were under his care died each day of diseases that are linked to diet. Kizer's official body count for an average day, from 1986 to 1991, included 193 dead of heart disease, 127 from cancer, 41 from stroke, and the rest from other assorted diet-related diseases.

Like Demopoulis, who has counseled such celebrities as Clint

Eastwood and Sylvester Stallone, Kizer virtually begged people to eat more fruits and vegetables (thought to protect against cancer). In fact, "Five [servings] a day for better health"—a campaign implemented by Kizer—has become a slogan up and down the coast of California. Kizer and others stress that although five servings of fruits and vegetables a day is acceptable, eight or nine servings is optimal.

California's numbers, which have remained steady, are graphic examples of a death toll that is sweeping the entire nation. Heart disease is the nation's number one killer, followed by cancer and stroke. If you add in diabetes and atherosclerosis (a thickening and hardening of the walls of the arteries, accompanied by small nodules of fatty substances), there are five diet-related causes of death among the country's top ten killers.

In 1991, *Longevity* magazine reported that two out of three deaths in this country are simply due to bad habits such as poor diet, excessive alcohol consumption, and tobacco use. Other experts have also cited such optimistic numbers. I say optimistic because if the deaths are due to bad habits, that means we have some real control over the situation.

The 1988 *Surgeon General's Report on Diet and Health,* a landmark declaration, attributed a full 35 percent of cancer deaths to diet, especially cancers of the colon, breast, and prostate. "That means 35 out of every 100 cancer deaths may have been avoided with a healthier diet," stressed Linda Dahl, a registered dietitian and past president of the California Dietetic Association, after studying the report.

Dr. Ernst Wynder, head of the American Health Foundation, a New York-based cancer research center, forty years ago was among the first scientists to prove a link between smoking and lung cancer. His current studies involve dietary fat and cancer, and he says about half of all cancers are related to fat in the diet. Edward L. Bierman, a professor of medicine and head of the division of metabolism endocrinology and nutrition at the University of Washington School of Medicine in Seattle, as well as the editor of *Good Health in Practice: Rx Nutrition,* has gone on record, along with the United States Department of Health and Human Services, as saying that diet plays a role in 70 percent of all deaths.

So, where's the optimism? What can be done? Noted nutrition

visionary John Robbins, son of the co-founder of Baskin-Robbins, the country's largest ice cream parlor chain, is also one of the country's biggest critics of beef and dairy products. He has been nominated for a Pulitzer Prize for one of his best-selling books on vegetarianism. When testifying during a government hearing on nutrition, he said that 97 percent of heart attacks could be prevented by a vegetarian diet. Demopoulis believes that changing one's diet can cut one's risk of certain cancers by 80 percent.

And just how many people are involved when we say heart disease is the country's number one killer, or cancer falls right behind it at number two? It's easy to say something affects a large number of people, but how many living, breathing Americans does that include? When the Department of Health and Human Services reported on such tragedies in 1990, the figures stated that 42,330,000 Americans were affected by heart disease, 37,000,000 by high blood pressure, 11,000,000 by diabetes, 4,640,000 by cancer, and 1,830,000 by strokes.

IT'S WHAT YOU'RE NOT EATING THAT MAY BE IMPORTANT

And just where do all those ominous numbers leave you? I hope you and your loved ones are not among those afflicted by these devastating diseases. The good news, of course, is that even if you already have certain diseases, like some forms of heart disease and high blood pressure, you can greatly improve—or reverse—your situation by modifying your diet. I also hope your name isn't on a recent roll sheet of 21,000 people surveyed by the United States Department of Agriculture. Believe it or not, not one person of the 21,000 questioned was getting the recommended daily allowances (RDAs) of ten nutrients (including vitamin C, water, calcium, iron, and fiber) needed for basic good health. And RDAs are the *bare minimum* requirements to stop you from becoming seriously ill. They are by no means the optimal amounts of nutrients for which to shoot.

That survey illustrates an important point. It's just as often essential, when it comes to disease prevention, to look at what you're *not* eating as it is to examine unhealthful eating habits (like eating too much dietary fat). And there are plenty of people keeping tabs on what you are not necessarily eating. The *American Journal of Public Health,* for example, reported that on an average day, 40 percent of Americans eat no fruit, 20 percent pass up all vegetables, and over 80 percent go without whole-grain breads or high-fiber grains and cereals. A survey reported by the *Fort Lauderdale News & Sun Sentinel* reported that, for some reason or another, 14 percent of those who make over $100,000 a year never eat any breakfast. The California Dietetic Association is alarmed because, although the state is a bountiful agricultural area, on any given day about a third of the state's residents eat no vegetables and half eat no fruit.

Another reason we're often not getting enough nutrients is our nation's concern with weight control. Many dieters are reading food labels to avoid certain components in food. James Heimbach, Ph.D., head of consumer research at the FDA's Center for Food Safety and Nutrition, calls this "single-issue dieting." For example, a dieter singles out sodium, cholesterol, or fat and avoids it. However, dieters must be careful. Research from the United States Department of Agriculture showed, for example, that women who, between 1985 and 1986, lowered fat and cholesterol in their diets often also lowered their daily intake of iron, calcium, and zinc.

YOU MAY NOT BELIEVE WHAT YOU ARE EATING

Although many of us try to ensure our health by avoiding certain foods, we may be eating some foods—or even non-foods—unwittingly. For example, let's say you get up one morning and decide to whip up a protein shake made with fresh orange juice and other ingredients. Would you first grab your kitchen garbage bag and swirl around a handful of garbage in the blender before blending your shake?

Unfortunately, that kind of thing seems to happen on a much larger scale. Some trucks that haul garbage have subsequently hauled food without even being cleaned. Also, in the United States it is not illegal to haul chemicals in a truck and then haul food. But it is illegal to contaminate food. Some food processing workers in Washington recently noticed a funny smell in a truck-load of orange juice concentrate. Upon inspection, a layer of thick, black chemical residue was found inside the tanker.

And what about after products are packaged? Can those small toys found in some cereals and other products affect the food? Can plastic trays in cookie or candy boxes have any effect?

Apparently, they sometimes produce offensive odors that consumers detect. The United States Food and Drug Administration has also voiced some concern that these extra items within the package may be the source of unwanted substances in foods.

You may also be eating insects without knowing it. I was surprised by an Associated Press report that stated, "Most Americans would not knowingly include insects, rodent hairs, or maggots in their daily diet, but they may be surprised to learn that these vermin and their residues may be in the food they eat." A seven-ounce glass of tomato juice, for example, can, under government standards, contain up to twenty fly eggs. A one-pound box of macaroni can have up to nine rodent hair fragments; 3.5 ounces of apple butter can have up to five whole insects; and a pound of cocoa beans can have up to ten milligrams of rodent feces. The FDA says these standards are acceptable and not harmful to health. However, I still think—whether it's rodent feces in your hot chocolate or garbage residue in your orange juice—that this is one more reason to be aware of what you are eating and to consciously try to eat better. There is not much we can do about unsanitary food conditions. But, if we are eating the most healthful diet possible, we are building our immune systems and are in better shape to handle such assaults.

A TASTE OF HOW FOOD CAN WORK FOR YOU

We've taken a preliminary look at the negative side of the picture—how eating too much of the wrong foods or not nearly enough of the right foods can make you very sick. But let's also briefly preview some of the newest findings regarding what great things eating nutritious foods can do for you.

- Researchers at Wynder's American Health Foundation recently made worldwide news by finding that a low-fat diet boosts immunity. Cutting fat in the diet can be associated with a rise in what Wynder calls "natural disease-killing cells," which possibly go and knock out viruses and cancerous cells.

- If you already have some form of atherosclerosis (fatty deposits in the arteries), switching to low-fat foods can slow the growth of new deposits. Obviously, if you don't have atherosclerosis, eating low-fat foods can help keep you from developing fatty deposits.

- A new study has shown that eating quite a bit of foods containing vitamin E early in life may help you avoid Parkinson's disease later. After studying 106 Parkinson's patients, Dr. Lawrence Golbe, a neurologist at the University of Medicine and Dentistry of New Jersey, found that those with the disease were less likely to have eaten foods high in vitamin E in their youth. Golbe had done a previous survey, which showed that people free of Parkinson's had eaten a lot of vitamin E-rich foods, such as peanuts and peanut butter.

- A recent study reported in the *American Journal of Clinical Nutrition* showed that when people whose diets contained high percentages of fat ate canned beans, their cholesterol levels were lowered.

- Intestinal polyps can become cancerous. Surgery is often needed to remove them. However, a 1990 study in New York showed that eating two servings of bran cereal a day can help shrink the polyps, sometimes so much that patients no longer need surgery. Eighty percent of participants with polyps were helped. Also, people prone to polyps who ate the cereal developed fewer of them than did participants in other therapies.

These are just a few examples of some new research regarding what good nutrition can do for you. Later, we'll look at some specific plans of action for avoiding the most dreaded diet-related diseases. In the meantime, maybe just some good-spirited competition can drive you onward. Shortly before this book was written, that corporate symbol "Poppin' Fresh," the Pillsbury Doughboy, appeared at photo opportunity after photo opportunity, blowing out birthday candles and granting countless interviews. It seems he had achieved incredible longevity for an advertising symbol: He had made it to twenty-five years. That's got to be at least one hundred in human years. He's obviously fit, as he's been in 611 commercials, comprising airtime of 16,200 minutes, has had his stomach poked 32,500 times, and has had his picture appear on product packages 25.4 billion times. So, live up to the challenge: Eat well. Don't let ''Poppin' Fresh'' be the only one to achieve longevity.

2

Heart Disease

Perhaps some things in life are meant to be mysteries. Unfortunately, one mystery involving health and nutrition is whether a person is suffering from heart disease. This is so much of a mystery that about 25 percent of all people who have a heart attack have sudden death as their first and only symptom.

Heart disease is by far this country's number one killer. If everyone set an alarm clock tonight for tomorrow morning's wake-up buzz, about 900 people would sleep through their wake-up call. That's how many people die of heart disease in an average eight-hour period—one every thirty-two seconds.

By the age of sixty, one in five men will have heart trouble. One in seventeen women has heart trouble by the same age. Look around a crowded shopping mall or ballpark or perhaps even your own large family reunion. Unfortunately, statistics show that many of those people will develop—or may already have developed—heart disease.

Don't think your age or sex will protect you against heart disease. The famed and long-term Framingham (Massachusetts) Heart Study shows that about 45 percent of all heart attack victims are under age sixty-five, and 5 percent are under age forty. In fact, some studies have shown that healthy adults under sixty-five have a 50-percent chance of suffering a heart attack if they have just two of the following risk factors: High cholesterol level, obesity, smoking, inactivity, high blood pressure. Many women are shocked to learn that heart disease is the leading cause of death among women. Heart attacks are sometimes thought to happen much more to men, but of the 540,000 Americans who die each year of heart disease, 250,000 are women.

About one-third of all adult Americans are at high risk for heart disease and need to balance their blood cholesterol, according to a recent study from the National Center for Health Statistics. And children are at risk, too. As many as two-thirds of all children have cholesterol levels higher than desirable, and 10 to 15 percent have levels high enough to put them at immediate risk.

Dr. Gerald Berenson, a Louisiana State University Medical Center researcher who heads the nation's largest study of heart disease in children, says screenings could predict about 60 percent of the children who will have heart disease as adults. They could then, at an early age, alter habits that might lead to or worsen the condition. Berenson says children, like adults, should be screened for such factors as blood pressure, cholesterol, weight, body fat, and family history. His findings stem from a study of about 10,000 people.

JUST WHAT IS CHOLESTEROL?

Obviously, high cholesterol isn't choosy. It will target your infant son, your elderly mother, or you. It is one of the three major risk factors for heart disease. (Smoking and high blood pressure are the others.) But just what is cholesterol? What is heart disease? What is a heart attack? Statistics of the skyrocketing incidences of heart disease, high cholesterol, and related problems make for interesting and scary reading. But often they leave out the "heart"of the picture: What's really going on inside you. Buying any of the plethora of food products available marked "no choles-terol" does nothing to tell you why you're trying to avoid choles-terol in the first place. Often, when that chilling scenario becomes vivid, so does the desire to control your risk factors.

Cholesterol is a soft, fat-like substance that gathers with the fats in the blood stream. It can be a culprit in the development of diseases of the heart and the blood vessels. However, cholesterol is manufactured in the body and also plays many important roles.

It is also present in all meat, fish, and dairy products. When we eat a lot of those foods, our blood cholesterol level can rise. As cholesterol builds up on their inner lining, blood vessels can narrow or even close. When that happens, oxygen-carrying blood is kept from getting to the heart or the brain. The eventual result can be severe chest pain or heart attack. The American Heart Association, as well as experts like Berenson, stress that atherosclerosis (the narrowing of the arteries) can begin in childhood and progress through young adulthood.

That's why it's important to keep your blood cholesterol, also referred to as serum cholesterol, at a safe level. The National Institutes of Health considers that number to be under 200 milligrams per deciliter (mg/dl). Some sources recommend even lower levels. An ideal level is said to be your age plus 100. That would make the 200 mg/dl an ideal number for 100-year-olds! It's important to remember that, as with the recommended daily allowances for nutrients, these guidelines are often written for the masses, not the individual who wants to reach optimal glowing health. Generally, 200 to 239 mg/dl is considered borderline-high serum cholesterol, and 240 mg/dl and above is high.

WHAT IS HEART DISEASE?

The heart works a lot like a pump pushing water through a garden hose. It is a large, fist-shaped muscle. Perhaps if it really were a fist it would take a good, hard swing at the culprits who blow smoke around it or feed it fatty foods. The heart, though, is busy enough already, of course. According to the American Health Assistance Foundation (AHAF), the average heart each day beats about 100,000 times and pumps about 2,000 gallons of blood.

According to AHAF coronary heart disease research, almost all Americans, even people in their twenties and some children, show signs of atherosclerosis, the hardening of the arteries. And atherosclerotic plaque has clearly been shown to be related to a fat-rich diet. That's why researchers recommend a diet that limits fat to 25 to 30 percent (or less) of caloric intake. Many Americans get as much as 40 percent of their calories from fat.

When a person's arteries are narrowed by atherosclerotic plaque, the heart can often function fairly well when the body is at rest. But at any sign of exertion, chest pain might be felt. This is angina. Much angina can be controlled with medication; however, it is a warning sign that a person is at much greater risk for heart attack and that his or her arteries have narrowed.

WHAT IS A HEART ATTACK?

A heart attack, also called a myocardial infarction, occurs when the blood supply to part of the heart muscle is severely reduced or stopped. This happens when either of the two coronary arteries, which supply blood to the heart, is blocked by an obstruction (or is narrowed, such as by the build-up of plaque and cholesterol). There are massive heart attacks and minor ones. Some people can have a heart attack without even knowing it. But any heart attack, whatever its severity, will leave part of the heart scarred and dead.

GET KNOWLEDGEABLE

It's the thesis of this book that it is definitely better to be scared than scarred, and it's certainly better to be scared than dead. With the huge numbers of people affected by heart disease in this country, being scared is justified. But my philosophy is: Don't get scared, get knowledgeable. Take precautions. Cut the fat in your diet. And don't think that heart disease can't happen to you.

For example, a recent study looked at 3,220 people age forty and up who showed no sign of cardiovascular disease. But with echocardiography, a type of ultrasound, 16 percent of the men and 21 percent of the women were shown to have an enlarged left ventricle, the heart's main pumping chamber. Over just four years, those with enlargements—even though they had shown no signs of heart disease—were shown to have a higher risk of developing and dying from the disease. In fact, every 40-percent increase in the heart muscle mass doubled the risk of dying, according to Dr. Daniel Levy of the Framingham Heart Study.

And just what caused this increase in the size of the left ventricle? Were the subjects born that way? According to Levy, that's not the case. The extra workload on the muscle from obesity and high blood pressure may cause the enlargement. What came out of the study is that echocardiography may be a much better indicator of enlarged ventricles than the much more commonly-used electrocardiograms, which detect the problem in only 1 percent of the people. But sometimes what comes out of these studies is much simpler. For example, the enlargement can be reversed by treating hypertension and losing weight.

TIPS ON DIET AND HEART DISEASE PREVENTION

Can changing the diet really help prevent disease? As all of the studies written about in this book scream from these pages: YES. A study of almost 13,000 men showed that dietary changes are even better than medication in preventing heart disease and other problems. The study, called the Multiple Risk Factor Intervention Trial, involved twenty-two centers across the country following the progress of the men for over ten years. The study was reported in the *Journal of the American Medical Association.*

A group of men at high risk for cardiac disease cut their chances of dying from a heart attack by 24 percent by changing to a low-fat, low-cholesterol diet. Each man in the study had two or more risk factors for heart disease but no obvious symptoms. Half received standard medical care, including either observation or drugs. The rest learned to eat better. After ten and a half years, a follow-up showed that the group that changed their diet had 10.6 percent fewer deaths from heart disease, 8.3 percent fewer deaths from cardiovascular disease, and 7.7 percent fewer deaths from other causes. Marcus Kjelsberg, the director of the study, said the researchers expect to see benefits when the men are given their fifteen-year follow-up, in 1996.

But why should you wait that long to find out such results? Get them for yourself starting right now. Following is some important information, adapted from the American Heart Association as well as the latest research, that you can use to trim the fat—and, therefore, the heart disease risk—from your diet.

- *Milk.* Two glasses of whole milk have 16 grams of fat; two servings of skim milk have just 2 grams of fat; non-fat milk has less than 1 gram.

- *Pizza.* One slice of pizza with a meat topping averages 12 grams of fat; one slice of pizza with vegetable toppings averages 5 grams of fat.

- *Bread.* One croissant has about 12 grams of fat; one dinner roll (choose whole-grain, if possible) has just 2 grams.

- *Meat.* One ounce of bologna has 8 grams of fat; one ounce of lean, broiled ham has just 1.5 grams.

With the guidelines throughout this book, you should also have all the tools available to accomplish the following tasks, which the American Heart Association, the American Dietetic Association, and others recommend for "heart health":

- Total fat intake should be less than 30 percent of daily calories. The latest research tells you to shoot for about 20 percent or less.

- Saturated fat should be less than 10 percent of daily calories.

- Polyunsaturated fat should not exceed 10 percent of daily calories.

- Cholesterol should not exceed 300 milligrams per day. Eat no more than two egg yolks per week, including those used in cooking.

- Carbohydrate intake should make up 50 percent or more of daily calories. Strive for mostly complex carbohydrates (whole grains, fruits, and vegetables).

- Protein intake can provide the rest of the daily calories. But think in terms of lean protein. Tofu, for example, has no cholesterol and little saturated fat.

- Sodium intake should not exceed 3 grams (3,000 milligrams) per day. Read product labels for sodium content.

- A wide variety of foods and any supplementation needed (see Chapter 18) should be consumed to get a balance of nutrients.

More specifically, what does all this mean for adults? It can mean eating every day: Five or more servings of vegetables and fruits (bumped up to nine servings when trying to prevent cancer); six or more servings of starchy vegetables or whole-grain, no-sugar breads and cereals; two or more servings of low- or non-fat dairy products; no more than two servings of meat, poultry, fish, or seafood (you can substitute two or more servings of dried beans and peas); and, if desired, five 1-teaspoon servings of unsaturated fats and oils. Red meat should be limited to two servings per week. (Check with your physician for the special needs of children, adolescents, and pregnant women.)

Following are some assorted tips that may come in handy:

- Avoid deep-frying or pan-frying in excess oil. Instead, stir-fry meats and vegetables in minimal oil. Try low-fat cooking methods, such as broiling, poaching, and steaming.

- Throw out fatty drippings. Baste lean meats with wine; with unsalted, no-fat canned broth; or with tomato or fruit juice.

- Place lean meat on a rack when roasting, broiling, or braising.

- Cook foods in a non-stick skillet using vegetable cooking spray.

- Make a broth for soups and stocks lower in fat. Just chill, then skim off the fat. The same can be done with stews, casseroles, and sauces: chill first, and skim off the fat.

- Try non-fat or low-fat yogurt in your salad dressings or dips.

- Good choices when it comes to cheeses are hoop cheese, Farmer's cheese, and cheeses made with part-skim milk (such as mozzarella or ricotta cheese).

- Where possible, substitute unsaturated oils—including olive, canola, corn, soybean, and safflower—for saturated fats like butter and shortening.

- In cream sauces, use evaporated skim milk instead of heavy cream or whole milk.

Heart disease is this country's number one killer. But there are many things you can do to keep that killer locked up and away from your good health. Watch what you eat. Cut down on fat. Get to be good friends with your cholesterol count. It could be a matter of life and death.

3

Cancer

Popular comedienne Gilda Radner and popular actor Michael Landon, like millions of other people, became cancer death statistics. What is also unfortunate is that Radner and Landon, again like so many cancer patients, did not understand the cancer-diet connection until it was too late.

When already very ill, they both rushed to change what they admitted was a lifetime of questionable eating habits. Radner, as she wrote in *It's Always Something*, her posthumously-published autobiography, turned to macrobiotics, a vegetarian way of eating. Landon, as he told many of his interviewers, hurriedly switched to a nutritionist-recommended vegetable- and fruit-based diet.

While virtually no one in the medical community will tell you that food will cure cancer, virtually everyone in that same community at this point recommends diet—the kind Radner and Landon and so many cancer patients grasp at much too late—as one of the best ways to *prevent* cancer from occurring in the first place.

The same week that mountains of articles were being printed about Landon's choice of treatment, three major studies were released that added to the tremendous amount of information that shows certain dietary choices are likely to help prevent cancer.

The Federation of American Societies for Experimental Biology released studies that showed eating more vegetables and less red meat can help reduce the risk of cancer. One of the studies was announced by Harvard Medical School researcher Edward Giovan-nucci and involved over 7,000 men between ages forty and seventy-five. Those who ate much less red meat than the others and increased their vegetable intake (which translated into a low-fat, high-fiber diet) were 33 to 50 percent less likely to develop polyps leading to colon cancer than were men who ate a high-fat, low-fiber diet.

The second study, also released by the Federation of American Societies for Experimental Biology, was of 500 men, half of whom had cancer of the larynx. Research showed that those who did not eat many vegetables were twice as likely to have gotten the cancer than those who ate a lot of vegetables. Those who had eaten high-fat diets were two and a half times as likely to have developed the cancer.

The third study released that week—this one by researchers at Tufts University—dealt with the finding that wheat bran topped rice bran, corn bran, barley bran, soy bran, and even oat bran as a possible prohibitor of colon cancer. (Each of those brans has spawned lots of research backing its own effectiveness.)

Despite these and other studies, many of us don't follow the medical community's advice until we've been felled by a deadly diagnosis. And when it comes to cancer prevention, that advice has been pouring in almost daily.

For instance about the time Landon announced his diagnosis, the Physicians' Committee for Responsible Medicine made news when it requested that the "four basic food groups" be changed from meat, fruits and vegetables, dairy products, and bread and cereal to whole grains, vegetables, legumes, and fruit. The group said there has been an overemphasis on protein and that, if they want to prevent disease, most Americans should cut their eating of animal protein by at least half.

Also started the month of Landon's diagnosis was a national campaign to get consumers to eat at least five servings of fruit and vegetables a day to prevent cancer. As mentioned earlier, however, many people eat almost no fruits and vegetables at all!

JUST WHAT IS CANCER
AND HOW MAY DIET PLAY A ROLE?

About 1,040,000 people in the United States will be diagnosed with cancer this year. About 510,000 people will die from it this year. Nearly 30 percent of Americans now living will have cancer at some point in their lives, and three of every four families will eventually be affected by the disease.

Any organ in the body can be the starting point for cancer. Cancer is an abnormal and uncontrolled growth of cells. As cancer spreads, normal cell division does not occur, and tumors build up. Tumors can be benign. When a malignant tumor is present, that is cancer. Malignant tumors can spread to other tissues and organs.

"No one knows for sure how a normal cell becomes a cancer cell," former National Cancer Institute director Vincent DeVita reported in the results of a cancer prevention awareness study. "But scientists agree that people get cancer mainly through repeated or long-term contact with one or more cancer-causing agents called carcinogens."

If those carcinogens happen to be in foods you enjoy daily, you are certainly fulfilling the cancer-promoting requirement that involves repeated or long-term exposure. And if you don't change your eating habits now, perhaps because you're waiting to see what new research regarding cancer and diet is completed in a few years, you just may be giving cancer a green light for growth. That's because almost all cancers develop slowly, appearing anywhere between five and forty years after the repeated exposure to risk factors.

Those risk factors can eventually become agents of cancer. Some agents seem to initiate cancer. Harvard researchers have shown, for example, that the probable role that animal fat plays in development of cancer of the colon is that it increases stomach bile, which then promotes tumors. Other agents seem to promote already-existing malignancies. Many studies have shown that excess fat in the diet can do both.

Unfortunately, I could fill this entire book with studies that have linked certain eating habits with the possible initiation and promotion of cancer. (Some of the essential nuts and bolts—and carrots and cantaloupes—involved in eating to prevent cancer will be explained later in this chapter.)

All of the studies completed reflect one thing: The usually diverse scientific and medical community wholeheartedly agrees that certain foods and groups of foods are involved in cancer development. So why, then, don't people adjust their diets accordingly? Part of the problem is that the information is available, but it has not yet been taken to heart (or colon or pancreas) by a large segment of the population. A report from the American Cancer Society compares the current diet/nutrition situation with the mounting evidence it brought out against smoking a few decades ago:

"Cancer research is now at the point vis-a-vis diet and nutrition that it was with smoking thirty years ago. The American Cancer Society decided then that the evidence against smoking, although limited, was sufficient to justify warning the public about the potential dangers. We have similarly concluded now that the data linking diet and cancer is convincing enough to justify issuing some dietary guidelines. These are similar to background statements issued by the National Research Council of the National Academy of Sciences, and the National Cancer Institute."

TIPS ON DIET AND CANCER PREVENTION

When Dr. Mark Messina, Ph.D., ate at a national cancer organization's banquet following his speech to the group about what a major role diet plays in the development of disease, he had a nice big salad.

Ironically, though, Messina, program director at the National Cancer Institute and one of the country's top experts on diet and cancer prevention, said his dinner was a special order since the rest of the group—to whom he had just explained what a poor dietary choice red meat can be—dined on huge slabs of roast beef.

There are specific tips researchers like Messina give for those trying to eat to prevent cancer. Cancer is taking a devastating toll—much of it clearly diet-related—on this country. Keep in mind:

- Messina is a supporter of soy foods, like tofu, as substitutes for meat in the diet. Through the National Cancer Institute, he has reported studies showing that rats on a soy diet developed many fewer tumors than those on more traditional American diets. "Even with only a 5-percent addition of soy to their diets," Messina said, "there was a 50-percent decline in the number of breast tumors." That translates, Messina added, into just one eight-ounce serving of tofu or two cups of soy milk per day.

Many people are not familiar with the taste of soy foods. But, as co-author of Avery Publishing Group's *The Tofu Book: The New American Cuisine,* I can tell you the taste is great. We developed over 150 Americanized tofu recipes and devised ways to hide the tofu so that no one but the chef needs to know they are eating it!

- Usually the front page of *The New York Times* bears headlines like: "Earthquake Shakes Turkey; at least 600 believed dead"; or "G.O.P. sees House bank affair as big weapon for campaigns." Well, on March 15, 1992, the front page of *The New York Times* did bear those headlines. But to show how far food research into cancer and disease prevention has come, the front page also proclaimed, "Potent element to fight cancer seen in broccoli."

The article's lead paragraph stated, "Broccoli harbors what could be the most powerful anti-cancer compound ever detected, scientists say. Researchers at Johns Hopkins University School of Medicine have isolated an ingredient in broccoli that kindles the activity of critical enzymes in the cell known to help guard against tumors. Many natural and synthetic compounds have been identified that stimulate these protective enzymes, but the newly discovered chemical in broccoli is by far the most powerful inciter."

The researchers said that it will be many years before broccoli's potent cancer guard can be bottled in pill form, if at all, but that eating broccoli is undoubtedly a good plan for anyone hoping to help ward off cancer.

Other scientists had suspected the broccoli link and think its powerful cancer inhibitors may also be found in onions and other foods. Dr. Terrance Leighton, professor of biochemistry at the University of California at Berkeley, has done research that indicates the compound quercetin, which is in broccoli, red and yellow onions, grapes, and yellow Italian squash, may also help protect against cancer.

Quercetin is "one of the strongest anti-cancer agents known," Leighton was quoted as saying more than a year before the broccoli results became known. "Well-documented studies show that enthusiastic onion and broccoli eaters have a lower risk of certain cancers. Quercetin is a prime reason," Leighton said. (But be aware that white onions do not contain quercetin.)

In dozens of lab studies, quercetin has blocked initial cell changes that set the stage for cancer. Quercetin also, Leighton said, powerfully suppresses the proliferation of malignant cells that amass into a tumor.

- The American Cancer Society and other organizations have been saying for some time that for cancer prevention we should eat more vegetables from the cruciferous group—including broccoli, cabbage, spinach, Brussels sprouts, cauliflower, bok choy, kale, radishes, rutabagas, and turnips. Cruciferous vegetables are characterized by thick, water-storing stems and leaves. Whenever possible eat fresh vegetables, because they tend to be more packed with nutrients. Steaming vegetables preserves the nutrients. And steaming them in a microwave preserves even more nutrients than when you steam on a stovetop. If you are eating for cancer prevention, the U.S. Department of Agriculture and other groups recommend upping your daily intake of all fruits and vegetables to nine servings.

- A massive, ten-year, ongoing study of the lifestyles of more than a million Americans is strengthening the belief by scientists that diets low in fiber and high in fats are major contributors to the risk of cancer. The study, backed by the American Cancer Society, is comparing habits and checking causes of death of every participant. Data is already confirming these Cancer Society cancer prevention suggestions: Cut down on fat intake; eat more high-fiber foods; eat foods rich in vitamins A and C; eat sparingly of foods cured with salt, smoke, or nitrites; and don't drink alcohol, or drink it very moderately.

- Populations consuming adequate amounts of vitamin A have lower rates of cancer of the lung, esophagus, mouth, pharynx, and larynx. Animal studies have also shown that vitamin A can suppress the growth of tumors. One population study from the State University of New York at Buffalo compared the diets of 450 lung cancer patients with the diets of over 900 healthy people. The results showed that those with the lowest beta-carotene intake were 80 percent more likely to get lung cancer than those with the highest. Keep in mind the adage about eating an apple a day, but add to that a carrot a day as well. The difference between the high and low carotene intakes? It was the equivalent of one carrot a day!

Dark green and deep yellow vegetables and fruits are some of the best sources of beta-carotene—the substance the body uses to make vitamin A. Besides carrots, rich sources of beta-carotene include spinach, tomatoes, winter squash, sweet potatoes, pumpkins, papayas, cantaloupes, mangos, apricots, and watermelons.

- Epidemiological studies show that people whose diet is rich in vitamin C are less likely to get cancer, particularly of the stomach and esophagus, than people whose diet lacks vitamin C. Vitamin C has been shown to inhibit the formation of carcinogenic nitrosamines in the stomach. Rich sources of vitamin C are citrus fruits (oranges, grapefruits, lemons, tangerines), tomatoes and their juices, broccoli, bell peppers, kiwi fruits, melons, papayas, and strawberries.

- Fat intake has long been linked to heart disease risk. However, in recent years fat has also become more and more strongly linked to the development of cancers. Dr. Ernst L. Wynder, president of the American Health Federation and among the first researchers to discover the link between cancer and tobacco, estimates that half of all cancers in women and a third of all cancers in men are related to dietary fat.

"I believe the major cause of disease is excessive exposure to fat," Wynder said. "I believe our system was not developed to handle 100 grams of fat a day." (Yes, many people consume that much fat daily.)

Excluding common skin cancers, the incidence of colorectal cancer ranks second only to lung cancer in this country. Lots of data is beginning to be discovered about dietary fat's link to colorectal and bowel cancers. "I think people are well aware of the role of dietary fat and heart disease, but the data haven't been as strong with dietary fat and cancer," Stanford University epidemiologist Alice Whittemore, co-author of a five-year study of the Chinese, cancer, and diet, told the *Los Angeles Times*. "I think that's changing, though. The data are beginning to come in quite conclusively on large bowel cancers, that fat is an important factor. I think this is an important public health message."

A rate of colorectal cancer four to five times higher among Chinese-Americans than among Chinese living in China can be strongly linked to a diet high in saturated fats, Whittemore's group at Stanford and researchers at the University of Southern California reported in a study published in the *Journal of the National Cancer Institute*.

Similar results have also been reported linking dietary fat to increased breast cancer in women. Also, researchers from the Harvard School of Public Health found that men with the lowest fat intake (an average of 24 percent of calories from fat) had only half the rate of adenoma colon polyps, a common precursor of colon cancer, of men with the highest fat intake (averaging 41 percent of calories from fat, which is not much higher than what the average American eats daily).

- Red meat has also been linked in a massive study to colon cancer. A study of 88,751 women reported in the *New England Journal of Medicine* showed that eating beef, pork, or lamb as a main dish every day increases the risk of colon cancer. Other studies have also hinted at such a link. A possible reason for the cancer development is that animal fat may increase stomach bile and promote tumors.

  "The risk of colon cancer has a direct relation to the amount of red meat consumed, so one can receive the majority of benefits by reducing intake to, say, once or twice a week," said study director Dr. Walter Willett of the Harvard School of Public Health. Willett said that substituting poultry or fish reduced risk substantially. Eating vegetable-based meals cuts the risk even more and, as we'll see in Chapter 22, can even prevent cancer.

- Eat more high-fiber foods. Observations indicate that the incidence of colon cancer is low in populations whose diet is made up largely of unrefined food. Fruits, vegetables, whole grains, and legumes contain varying amounts of fiber and are unrefined. Refined carbohydrates (sugar, white flour, etc.) contain little or no fiber. Fiber is also absent from animal foods and fats.

The National Cancer Institute recommends that we eat about thirty to thirty-five grams of fiber a day (but not more than forty).

Low-fat, high-fiber diets are also associated with weight loss and weight maintenance. So follow the recommendations for cancer prevention and the tips in the preceding chapter on heart disease prevention, and you should lose any and all excess weight you may be carrying around.

4

Diabetes

Esther Miller, a Detroit housewife, had an active sweet tooth. She loved cookies, candy, and cake. Although she always promised herself she was going to cut down, she never managed to do so. When Miller was recently diagnosed with Type II diabetes, she remembered all of the times she had heard that eating a lot of sugar could cause diabetes. She was sure sugar must have caused her diabetes.

Actually, the notion that eating sugar causes diabetes is a myth. However, refined sugar, the ultimate empty-calorie food (at 2,500 calories per pound), can contribute to obesity, which is often a trigger for diabetes. Miller fit the prediabetic profile, not because she ate a lot of sugar, but because she tipped the scales at 280 pounds.

Miller joined the ranks of the more than 12 million people in the United States who have diabetes. About 10 million of them have Type II (non-insulin-dependent) diabetes. Significantly, more than 80 percent of those with Type II diabetes are overweight.

The precise cause of diabetes is still a scientific mystery. However, heredity seems to play a role. Obesity, though, seems to play just as significant a role. When one is genetically prone to diabetes, becoming obese can trigger the onset of Type II diabetes. Our cells need glucose (a type of sugar). Body fat can form a type of barrier that does not allow insulin (a hormone) to transport glucose into the cells.

Diabetes causes 125,000 to 150,000 deaths per year in the United States, where it is a leading killer and cause of blindness. Those with diabetes are three times more likely than others to suffer from heart disease. Diabetes and high blood pressure are also the main causes of kidney failure. "Many people don't know they have kidney damage, because they feel no pain and have experienced no change in urinary habits," the National Institute of Diabetes and Digestive and Kidney Diseases (a division of the United States Department of Health and Human Services) warned in an advisory.

"So strong is the link between Type II diabetes and obesity that some experts have blended the problems into a single term. Their chief weapon in fighting 'diabasity' is a nutritionally balanced weight loss diet," according to the *Mayo Clinic Nutrition Letter*.

The American Diabetes Association considers the following to be indicators of the possible onset of diabetes. Experiencing any of these symptoms on a regular basis should cause concern:

- excessive thirst
- frequent urination
- extreme fatigue
- unexplained weight loss
- blurry vision from time to time

In addition, answering yes to a number of the following statements can also indicate a proneness to diabetes:

- I am over forty years old.
- I am at least 20 percent over my ideal weight.
- I am a woman who has had more than one baby weighing over nine pounds at birth.
- I am of American Indian descent.
- I am of Latino or African-American descent.
- I have a parent with diabetes.
- I have a sibling with diabetes.

To contact the American Diabetes Association for pamphlets or other information, call (800) 232–3472.

By ignoring the warning signs of diabetes, you run the risk of developing other medical problems, too.

A study in the June 1990 issue of the *Journal of the American Medical Association* showed that people who develop diabetes have many signs of heart disease years before the diabetes symptoms appear. A team led by Dr. Michael Stern of the University of Texas Health Science Center in San Antonio followed over 600 Mexican-Americans (who historically have been more prone to diabetes) for eight years. Those who eventually developed diabetes were much more likely than the others to have had high blood pressure, high triglycerides (blood fat related to heart disease), and high blood insulin.

"To bring risk [of developing heart disease] down, you have to start early," said Stern. "If you wait until you already have diabetes, you may have waited too long."

The key, then, is prevention, by eating a diet that keeps weight, blood pressure, cholesterol, triglycerides, and blood insulin at normal levels. Unfortunately, many people wait until they get a diabetes diagnosis and only then radically change their diet. However, if those changes were made as a matter of prevention, such potentially deadly diseases as diabetes could possibly be side-stepped.

5

Hypoglycemia

If you pop a doughnut in your mouth or nibble on a few candy bars in the morning, you are probably not thinking about the commute you may have to make later to work, the stack of typing you'll have to do once you get there, or the lecture you are planning to attend that evening.

However, later when you are driving, typing, or trying to listen intently to a speaker, your body—specifically your brain, pancreas, liver, and adrenal glands—may very well remember that doughnut or candy break. That's because if you have hypoglycemia (low blood sugar) each of those organs plays a role. When you eat sugary foods like doughnuts and candy bars, your body can overreact, leading to low blood sugar, which can bring on fatigue as well as interfere with the concentration involved in trying to drive, type, or study.

A number of diseases can cause low blood sugar, but that type of low blood sugar—often called *reactive hypoglycemia*—is rare. What is not rare, however, is *functional hypoglycemia*, which can occur even if your organs are in good shape. Poor eating habits can cause functional hypoglycemia to develop. Hypoglycemia can also accompany *diabetes mellitus* (also referred to as "sugar diabetes"). Since fat can interfere with blood sugar regulation, obesity can also be a factor in hypoglycemia.

Normal blood sugar is usually about 80 to 90 milligrams of glucose per deciliter of blood (mg/dl) before eating and 120 to 130 mg/dl after eating. However, two to three hours after eating, the blood sugar of someone who suffers from hypoglycemia can drop to 40 mg/dl or less.

In *Dr. Crook Discusses Hypoglycemia*, Dr. William G. Crook explains sugar's relationship to hypoglycemia:

"Sugar is the main villain in functional hypoglycemia. . . . Sucrose is a double compound containing two molecules, one glucose and one fructose. These molecules are bound together by a single link. By contrast, in foods such as fruits, vegetables, and meats, glucose and other molecules are tied together in long chains. When you eat a good diet . . . glucose molecules are released gradually. And your body's cells run better because their fuel is supplied evenly.

"By contrast, when you eat sweets (sucrose), enzymes from your small intestines break the bonds between the glucose and fructose molecules and glucose surges into your blood stream. And your blood glucose goes up like a jet-propelled missile. . . . If you keep eating sweets and other refined carbohydrates, your pancreas may overreact. And it puts out too much insulin, causing your blood sugar to drop to abnormally low levels. This makes you nervous, tired, and hungry. And your body craves sugar. . . . But when you eat sweets, you relieve your symptoms for only a short time. And your blood sugar goes up and down like a yo-yo."

Doctors offer tests for hypoglycemia. However, hypoglycemia is one condition that many experts suggest you can test for, to some extent, by yourself. If you crave sweets, and experience headaches, depression, fatigue, or irritability after eating them, you may want to try your own test. Simply stop eating refined sugar and refined (enriched) carbohydrates. That includes candy and cake and enriched breads and pastries. Instead of eating three big meals or skipping meals and eating irregularly, eat four to six smaller meals throughout the day.

If after following this program for a week you feel a lot better and lose some weight, you may have a good indication—without having taken expensive tests—that a hypoglycemic diet may be of benefit to you. And besides, experts stress, this type of diet (which features whole, fresh, unrefined foods, including vegetables, whole grains, and lean meat or protein) is the kind all of us concerned with our health should be striving for anyway!

6

Weight Gain

It certainly looked convincing when talk show superstar Oprah Winfrey wheeled sixty-seven pounds of simulated fat onto her show's stage in front of millions of television viewers. It also looked convincing when Winfrey ripped off a bulky outfit she was wearing to reveal the new body she had squeezed into a pair of size eight Calvin Klein jeans. All of this was, in fact, so compelling that hundreds of thousands of those viewers immediately clogged the telephone lines of the liquid diet beverage company she identified as a partner in her obvious weight loss.

Clearly, multimillionaire Winfrey is a powerful and persuasive woman. I met her in November 1989 when I was reporting on a seminar in which she was giving her tips for success. Dozens of women stood up at that sold-out seminar and told trim Winfrey how she had inspired them to go on the same diet she had. Many had lost significant amounts of weight.

If their goal, however, was to emulate Winfrey, then many of them might now be careening up and down a nightmarish diet roller coaster. That's what happened to Winfrey. In November 1989, she was very slim. By March 1990, *USA Today* was still praising her. They said her having regained seventeen pounds still left her ahead of most dieters. Within a few months, however, Winfrey had put back virtually all of the weight she had lost. In a *People* magazine cover story that seemed a bit more like public relations damage control than genuine sentiment, the headline said that Winfrey, "chubby again, drops dieting and develops a new attitude toward carrying her weight."

Winfrey has admitted she never learned to eat a nutritious diet. She drank weight-loss protein drinks and exercised to lose weight but soon afterward gave up the exercise and went back to a diet of fried, greasy foods and sweets. In her own words, she reverted to "eating like a pig." As unique and successful as Winfrey is, when it came to the weight-loss battle, she became just another casualty, another statistic.

ARE YOU PART OF AMERICA'S OVERWEIGHT CROWD?

Even if we didn't count the thousands of overweight people Winfrey probably influenced through her television show, she would still have lots of company in that battle. One in four people in the United States is overweight. Of these approximately 60 million people, over 12 million are severely overweight. Weight Watchers surveys show that 40 percent of all adults are trying to lose weight. In those surveys, women said that they want to lose an average of twenty-five pounds; men, an average of thirty-six pounds.

Overweight is usually defined as 20 percent over ideal weight, as identified by life insurance charts. (See Table 6.1 on page 41.) These charts have to do with correlations between overweight and mortality rates. Obesity—the state of being severely overweight—is generally considered being 40 percent above the recommended weight for one's height and build. Of course, there are variations on this theme. An overweight person who is active may have a significant amount of muscle rather than fat, thereby decreasing the health risk. A number on a scale can never tell the whole story.

Even if you are not severely or moderately overweight now, you might still be headed in that direction. The average American adult gains one pound per year, according to the American Dietetic Association. That adds up to about a thirty-pound weight gain between young adulthood and middle age.

Many people think that weight gain occurs more frequently with aging. Often, though, that is not the case. A 1990 Centers for

Table 6.1. Ideal Weights for Men and Women
Age Twenty-Five and Over*

	Men		
Height	Weight (lbs) for Small Frame	Weight (lbs) for Medium Frame	Weight (lbs) for Large Frame
5'2"	112–120	118–129	126–141
5'3"	115–123	121–133	129–144
5'4"	118–126	124–136	132–148
5'5"	121–129	127–139	135–152
5'6"	124–133	130–143	138–156
5'7"	128–137	134–147	142–161
5'8"	132–141	138–152	147–166
5'9"	136–145	142–156	151–170
5'10"	140–150	146–160	155–174
5'11"	144–154	150–165	159–179
6'0"	148–158	154–170	164–184
6'1"	152–162	158–175	168–189
6'2"	156–167	162–180	173–194
6'3"	160–171	167–185	178–199
6'4"	164–175	172–190	182–204

	Women		
Height	Weight (lbs) for Small Frame	Weight (lbs) for Medium Frame	Weight (lbs) for Large Frame
4'10"	92–98	96–107	104–119
4'11"	94–101	98–110	106–122
5'0"	96–104	101–113	109–125
5'1"	99–107	104–116	112–128
5'2"	102–110	107–119	115–131
5'3"	105–113	110–122	118–134
5'4"	108–116	113–126	121–138
5'5"	111–119	116–130	125–142
5'6"	114–123	120–135	129–146
5'7"	118–127	124–139	133–150
5'8"	122–131	128–143	137–154
5'9"	126–135	132–147	141–158
5'10"	130–140	136–151	145–163
5'11"	134–144	140–155	149–168
6'0"	138–148	144–159	153–173

*Table shows height in shoes and weight in indoor clothing.

Disease Control (CDC) study that tracked 10,000 adults age twenty-five to seventy-four for a decade showed that major weight gains of thirty pounds or more occurred most often in the youngest age group, who were twenty-five to thirty-four years old. Also likely to have a major weight gain were those thirty-four to forty-four years old.

Watch out, the study reported, because "middle-age spread" often begins well before middle age. In fact, your "fat wheels" may be in motion at any age, even before you ever see the outer bulges. "Becoming fat and being fat are two different phenomena, although people tend to focus on the aftermath," David Williamson, the CDC epidemiologist who led the study, told the *Los Angeles Times.*

OVERWEIGHT KIDS: EXPLODING NUMBERS NOW, EXPLODING ARTERIES IN THE FUTURE?

Research has shown that today's typical children are sedentary, unfit, and overweight. They are most comfortable sitting in front of a television set or a video game. Processed junk food is being consumed in increasing quantities. The bleak result is an alarming escalation of obesity in children.

A report by Harvard University's Department of Behaviorial Science showed that in the past two decades obesity has increased 54 percent among six-to-eleven-year-olds and 39 percent among twelve-to-seventeen-year-olds. Other surveys have shown that since 1983, the average weight of boys age ten to eighteen has increased by fourteen pounds.

A child doesn't have to eat huge quantities of food to gain weight. An extra 200 calories a day, the Mayo Clinic Nutrition Letter reminds parents, can cause a child to gain about half a pound a week. Those 200 calories could come from eating as seemingly innocent a snack as four homemade chocolate chip cookies.

According to the President's Council on Physical Fitness and Sports, because of poor diet, 40 percent of all American children between the age of five and eight show at least one of these heart disease risk factors: Obesity, elevated cholesterol, and high blood pressure. Studies also show that most overweight kids become overweight adults.

OVERWEIGHT: THE RISKS

We often hear that being overweight or obese increases a person's risk of developing high cholesterol levels, high blood pressure, heart disease, cancer, and diabetes. However, we have heard those words so many times that they may have lost their impact. So let's take a look at what excesss body weight actually does inside our bodies. This can be a much more graphic deterrent than would a shopping list of the diseases to which we may eventually succumb.

First of all, regardless of how much food they may be eating, most overweight people actually suffer from borderline malnutrition. Often, the food being consumed does not provide the optimal—or even the minimal—amounts of vitamins or minerals needed for good health.

We have heard a lot about fat cells. But how many fat cells do you have in your body? An average person has 30 to 40 billion fat cells. An obese person may have 180 billion.

Don't think you can't get rid of fat cells. You can with weight loss. You can also add lots of fat cells at any point in your life if you gain weight. There are a number of accepted theories concerning fat cells.

Fat is stored both in regular body cells and in special fat cells. For many years, the accepted theory was that the number of fat cells in an individual's body is determined early and remains the same throughout life. Further, it was believed that, once created, fat cells would always remain full of fat.

But as Helen Guthrie points out in *Introductory Nutrition*, a widely-used textbook in medical and nutrition schools, scientists have now discovered that the truth is more complicated than that. "We now know that the number of fat cells can increase in adult life and that the number of fat cells can also actually diminish as the result of sustained weight loss," she writes. Still, while it is possible to decrease the total number of fat cells in the body, there is evidence that people who have a large number of them will have a harder time keeping their weight down. Guthrie says this seems to be because "they seem to be able to lose weight up to the point where cell size reaches a 'normal level' but because of the larger number of cells, it is difficult to reduce beyond that point."

To gain one pound of weight, you must eat 3,500 more calories than you burn. Therefore, to lose one pound a week, you need to eat 500 fewer calories a day than you burn. Any excess calories will be turned into fat. Here's how:

Carbohydrates that are not immediately broken down into glucose are stored as glycogen. Glycogen is an insoluble starch-like substance in tissue. The body can convert it into sugar when necessary. The cells that store the glycogen can only hold so much of it. Any overflow is changed to fat and transported to fat cells. Much of the fat from foods is also sent for storage to fat cells. Excess protein is also changed into fat and stored. Unfortunately, as the *Mayo Clinic Nutrition Letter* points out, "Your body can store an unlimited amount of fat."

Although many of us hear the word "calorie" daily, just as many of us might very well flunk if we were asked to define the term on a pop quiz.

A calorie represents the units of energy (heat) contained in foods or alcohol. It is a means of measuring that energy. A kilocalorie (kcal) is the amount of heat required to raise the temperature of one kilogram of water by one degree Celsius. A calorie is equal to .001 kcal. Although kilocalorie and calorie have two distinct meanings, they are often used interchangeably, at times even in scientific literature.

So, now that we all understand what calories and kilocalories are, let's forget about them! Although a decade ago you probably wouldn't have caught many serious dieters without their portable food scales (which helped them monitor their caloric intakes), the prevailing wisdom from virtually everyone in the nutrition community today is that calories do not count nearly as much as other elements.

It is the quality of your overall diet that should be of concern to you, whether you are trying to maintain, gain, or lose weight. For example, you could keep your calorie count low by consuming daily, say, three diet sodas (3 calories), one of those "healthful" diet frozen dinners that might be full of additives and sugar (350 calories), and some coffee, tea, vegetables, and fruit. But calories are by no means the whole story.

You probably wouldn't have much energy if, like so many dieters, you ate that way. The key to weight loss is a high-fiber, low-fat diet. A number of studies have shown that those who eat such a diet lose more weight and lose it quicker than those eating lower-calorie foods filled with fat, additives, sugar, or artificial ingredients. High-fiber, low-fat foods, especially complex carbo-hydrates, are now known to be better fuels for your body. By planning your diet around these foods, you'll be able to lose weight *and* feel terrific—all the while knowing that you haven't sacrificed good nutrition in the bargain.

7

Eating Disorders

Celebrities appear regularly on television offering to show you how to lose weight. Weight loss centers, now on virtually every street corner in America, also launch exhaustive campaigns to teach the tricks of the trade for slimming down.

Of course, the celebrities who offer weight loss advice and the diet centers either don't realize or refuse to admit that they may be training you to acquire an eating disorder. They would argue that they are simply promoting weight loss—an important solution to a serious health problem in our society.

However, the American Dietetic Association and many other important nutrition groups warn that over 60 percent of people who have dieted extensively will resort to an eating disorder, like binging and purging, to try to keep the weight off. Unfortunately, some commercial diet organizations—and many stringent weight loss diets—are often the breeding ground for eating disorders. The poor nutrition habits that often accompany a desperate attempt to stay thin can become the jailer that keeps sufferers locked in the prison of an eating disorder.

WHO HAS EATING DISORDERS?

Over 75 percent of all United States women will experience some form of eating disorder at some point in their lives. Approximately

35 percent of all women college students practice some form of binge-and-purge behavior, whether it be full-fledged bulimia (gorging followed by vomiting), or gorging followed by starvation dieting, or gorging followed by compulsive exercising in an attempt at purging. Up to 10 percent of all young women will become anorexic (self-starvers), and each year 150,000 women die from that disorder.

As Naomi Wolf points out in her acclaimed book *The Beauty Myth,* if the 150,000 figure is true, then "every twelve months there are 17,024 more deaths [from anorexia] in the United States alone than the total number of deaths from AIDS tabulated by the World Health Organization in 177 countries and territories from the beginning of the epidemic through 1988" and "more die of anorexia in America each year than died in ten years of civil war in Beirut."

The pressure on men and boys to be slim and fit has also greatly increased in recent years. "Widespread practices to decrease weight and increase exercise can set off an eating disorder in vulnerable men," Dr. Arnold E. Andersen, director of the Eating and Weight Disorders Clinic at Johns Hopkins Hospital, told *The New York Times.*

In 1986, when I crisscrossed the country to promote my first book, *Biting the Hand That Feeds Me: Days of Binging, Purging and Recovery,* I was among the first guests to tell the huge audiences of "The Sally Jessy Raphael Show," "Hour Magazine," Cable News Network, and "Live With Regis and Kathie Lee" just what a tremendous toll eating disorders were taking on the young people of this country. At that point, although not new to the thousands experiencing such crises, the information was still new to the media and the general public.

I would have bet, however, that in the years since, as a flood of information and warnings were released, the incidence of eating disorders would decrease and not increase. I would have lost that bet. I always thought that the people of my generation (now approaching their thirties) would have avoided eating disorders had we known the potential dangers of participating in those strange rituals. But when I speak at high schools and junior high schools, I am still deluged with young women telling me that they or their friends are uncontrollably and miserably involved in such activities—even though they are aware of the dangers.

CAN WHAT YOU EAT (OR DON'T EAT) GIVE YOU AN EATING DISORDER?

Clearly, some eating disorders are not caused solely by the foods we eat or don't eat. In some cases, chemical imbalances or other physical problems bring on symptoms.

However, in most cases, diet is certainly a culprit. *USA Today* recently said in a headline: "One-third of girls are dieting, but most aren't fat." In fact, a recent study by the American Psychiatric Association (APA) found that 36 percent of girls age ten to twenty are dieting. In that study, 38 percent of girls and 49 percent of mothers told the APA they thought they were overweight and were taking measures to combat the perceived flab. The girls wanted to lose about ten pounds, and the mothers wanted to lose about twenty pounds. However, a full 70 percent of those in the survey were actually considered underweight by their physicians.

When people drastically reduce their calories to lose excess pounds that don't even exist, they are initiating a cycle they might not be able to control. Their metabolic rate, which determines how quickly or slowly they lose or gain weight, may slow down. A slowed metabolism makes each attempt at dieting tougher and makes it much easier to gain weight.

Drastic reductions in calories can also make people crave certain foods. If you are not eating enough food or getting enough nutrients, your body may send you strong signals that you'll perceive as the desire for certain foods. Almost all people with eating disorders are prey to these seemingly uncontrollable food cravings. Giving in to the craving for a large quantity of food is one of the first things that can force dieters onto a binge/purge roller coaster. They will eat a lot and then not eat at all to make up for it. This can become a habit that is almost impossible to break.

Many people need professional help to extricate themselves from an eating disorder. However, just about everyone involved in the field of health seems to agree that good nutrition is an essential component in treating eating disorders. "The key to treatment is to establish and maintain regular healthy eating habits," the Mayo Clinic has advised. "Skipping meals and fasting lead to eating binges."

Because of the partaker's food sensitivities, certain foods or substances in foods can trigger eating behaviors that lead to eating disorders. Refined sugar, caffeine, and enriched products are involved in some people's eating disorders. When these people avoid their problem substances, their eating desires become much more normalized.

Findings like this offer us some insight into the factors involved in eating disorders, although overcoming them is rarely that simple. Often there are complex emotional factors involved as well, and professional treatment may be necessary for recovery. But if you follow a natural, nutritious eating plan and avoid processed food as much as possible, you are likely to be many steps ahead when it comes to preventing eating disorders.

8

Osteoporosis

One day, seventy-two-year-old Mary Ingwald bent over to tie her shoe. Nine weeks later she was dead. Ingwald, who without being aware of it suffered from osteoporosis (brittle bones), fractured her hip while trying to tie her shoe. She was forced to enter a nursing home to recuperate. There, she developed pneumonia and died.

Ingwald's fifteen-year-old granddaughter, Heather Slater, knew that her grandmother's broken hip resulted from something called "osteoporosis." Although she had heard the word a number of times, she was not sure exactly what it meant. She thought it had something to do with elderly people. When asked if she drank any milk, Slater said she rarely did. Diet soda—about four cans a day—was her beverage of choice.

The late Ingwald and the young Slater are at two ends of the lifelong time line leading to osteoporosis. Can osteoporosis kill? Not directly, but complications from injuries due to the condition can. When young people like Heather Slater hit seventy-two, will it really matter if they drank milk or ate other calcium-rich products when they were fifteen? The answer, more and more research shows, is a resounding "yes."

We often lament that so many of the elderly end up in nursing homes. Did you know, though, that almost one-third of the women in nursing homes are there because of fractures? Eighty-five percent of those fracture victims are admitted because of a hip fracture, one of the main results of osteoporosis.

Mary Ingwald's situation was by no means rare. Drs. Cedric and Frank Garland explain in *The Calcium Connection* just what dire circumstances can occur: "The consequences are serious. This is because a broken hip often requires a period of immobilization, and immobilization can be deadly. Extensive time in bed can sometimes result in pneumonia or the development of blood clots, either of which can be fatal; a third of women will die within a year of an osteoporotic hip fracture."

JUST WHAT IS OSTEOPOROSIS?

Like Slater, many of us have heard the word "osteoporosis" lots of times. But how many of us know exactly what the condition is or how it can be easily prevented by acting early enough?

Osteo means bone, and *porosis* means increased pores. Increases in the bones' pores will eventually affect one in four United States women. Currently, almost 20 million women have osteoporosis. Some men also get osteoporosis, but it is more prevalent in women because of hormonal differences between the sexes and because women tend to have less bone mass to start with than men, who as a group are larger. Although the effects of osteoporosis usually show up in the middle-aged and the elderly, it cannot be stressed enough that the condition is set in motion many years earlier. Most importantly, it can be prevented during the years it is developing.

Like Ingwald, many people are unaware that they have osteoporosis until they suffer their first fracture. Osteoporosis gradually but continually depletes the mass of bones, which eventually become thin, fragile, and prone to fracture. A stooped posture called "dowager's hump," (a skeletal deformity for which there is no cure) and fractures of the spine, hips, and wrist are common. Bending over to tie a shoe, picking up a bag of groceries, or misstepping on a street curb may be all it takes to fracture bones made brittle by osteoporosis.

Some people are at higher risk than others. Answering yes to any of the following may put you at a higher risk:

- You are a white or Oriental female and have a petite or very thin body.

- You have had natural or surgical menopause before the age of forty-five.

- You have a mother or sister who had osteoporosis.

- You have not gotten adequate dietary calcium or exercise throughout your life.

- You smoke cigarettes.

- You drink more than two alcoholic beverages on a daily basis.

BONING UP ON BONE MASS INFORMATION

Calcium is essential every day to form and re-form the skeleton. There are 206 bones in the human body, and 99 percent of the calcium in our bodies at any given time is in our bones. The remaining calcium is in our blood.

Our bodies cannot manufacture calcium. The only way we can obtain it is by eating or drinking foods that contain calcium or, as a lesser option, taking calcium supplements. If we do not treat ourselves to enough calcium through our food to maintain the calcium in our blood, the body will pull stores of calcium from our bones.

There is an absolutely critical situation in this country regarding women and calcium. Almost 80 percent of all women do not get enough calcium. The body uses 500 to 550 milligrams of calcium each day. However, the average daily intake of calcium for women is about 490 milligrams, and 25 percent of women eighteen and older get less than 300 milligrams.

As the Garlands point out in *The Calcium Connection*, a deficiency like that can exact a toll. They estimate that about half of American women are losing bone throughout their adult lives:

"The condition is like a dripping faucet—the amounts involved are small, but they add up. You may lose only a few milligrams of bone a day, but this loss over several decades will leave you with a substantially reduced skeleton when you reach your sixties or seventies. If you lose 30 percent to 40 percent of your bone mass, your spinal column will gradually collapse."

The recommended daily allowance (RDA) of calcium for women age twenty-five and older is 800 to 1,000 milligrams, even though the body might use only 500 milligrams. That's because not all dietary calcium is absorbed. Vitamin D, which we can get from sunshine and other sources, also needs to be present. That's why milk, which is fortified with vitamin D, is a good calcium choice.

The RDAs are just guidelines. They call for males and females six months and younger to get 360 milligrams; six months to twelve months, 540 milligrams; one to ten years, 800 milligrams; eleven to twenty-four years, 1200 milligrams; after age twenty-four, 800 milligrams. However, those are just the minimums for good health. Many nutritionists suggest 1,000 milligrams after age twenty-four and 1,500 milligrams for post-menopausal women.

The good news is that bone loss can be reduced at any age if the diet is corrected. Many studies, including some at Tufts University that were reported in the *New England Journal of Medicine*, show that post-menopausal women who increase their formerly low calcium intake are able to reduce bone loss in their spines, hips, and forearms.

CRUCIAL EARLY PREVENTION

Although damage from osteoporosis can be reduced in later life, by far the most crucial time to take action is in the teen and young adult years.

Except during infancy, the body's greatest need for calcium is during adolescence. If, and only if, adequate calcium is supplied, bones continue to lengthen from age ten to nineteen. Did you know that the final size of our bones when we are about nineteen determines the amount of calcium that can be deposited in them? More calcium deposits reduce the chance of having weak bones later in life.

Young adults are lucky enough to still be at an age when they can add to their bone mass, for bones gain in density throughout a person's twenties and thirties. Through diet, people can increase their bone mass by as much as 20 percent during their critical young adult years.

High-protein and high-salt diets can interfere with the absorption of calcium in the body. So can certain favorite foods of teenagers, such as soda. Forgoing milk for soda, as Mary Ingwald's granddaughter Heather did, can mean a higher risk of osteoporosis later in life.

A 1990 Mayo Clinic study found that young women's typical diets—low in calcium and high in phosphorus from soft drinks and processed foods—may decrease the amount of bone they develop.

"The smaller the peak bone mass, or amount of bone present by around age thirty-five, the greater the chance of osteoporosis later in life," said Dr. Mona Calvo, who led the Mayo research. "Diet . . . can influence whether or not we reach full potential. This is particularly true for teens and young adults who are still building bone."

Calvo compared hormone and mineral levels of two groups of healthy women age eighteen to twenty-five. One group ate a diet with the recommended amounts of calcium and phosphorus. The other group ate half as much calcium and twice as much phosphorus. Calvo noted that the second group's diet closely matched that of average teens. Some of the foods they ate—sodas, processed cheese products, puddings—had phosphorus-containing food additives.

After four weeks, researchers noted changes in the hormone and mineral metabolism of the second group. When calcium intake is too low, the body usually springs into action by triggering mechanisms to conserve and better absorb calcium. The researchers were alarmed to find, however, that because of the excess phosphorus, this was not occurring. Their conclusion was that the young women studied, and the hundreds of thousands who eat similar diets, may not be able to achieve maximum bone mass. Previous studies have shown that caffeine-containing beverages can have the same effect on stunting bone mass.

SO WHAT CAN I EAT TO BOOST MY CALCIUM INTAKE?

You don't have to be a milk-lover to boost your calcium intake. Many vegetables have significant amounts of calcium. People who get much of their protein from vegetables—in this country and worldwide—have been shown to have much lower rates of osteoporosis.

Table 8.1. Calcium-Rich Foods

Food	Serving Size	Calcium Level (Milligrams)
Dairy		
Low-fat yogurt (plain)	1 cup	415
Low-fat yogurt (fruit-flavored)	1 cup	345
Skim milk	1 cup	302
Low-fat milk	1 cup	297
Whole milk	1 cup	291
Buttermilk	1 cup	285
Swiss cheese	1 ounce	272
Cheddar cheese	1 ounce	204
Cottage cheese (low-fat)	1 cup	154
Vegetables		
Collard greens	1 cup	335
Bok choy	1 cup	250
Roasted soynuts	½ cup	230
Turnip greens	1 cup	200
Kale	1 cup	200
Broccoli	1 cup	180
Soybeans	1 cup	175
Kelp (seaweed)	½ cup	170
Mustard greens	1 cup	150
Great Northern beans	1 cup	140
Vegetarian baked beans	1 cup	130
Kidney beans	1 cup	115
Other		
Sardines (canned with bones)	3 ounces	372
Oysters (raw)	1 cup	226
Soups made with milk	1 cup	168–191
Pink salmon (canned with bones)	3 ounces	167
Tofu (processed with calcium)	4 ounces	154

That's because diets high in animal protein can cause calcium depletion. According to Dr. Mark Messina, a program director of the National Cancer Institute's Diet and Cancer branch, vegetable-based diets do not have that effect. Because of this, vegetarians often can get by with eating less dietary calcium than those who eat a lot of animal protein.

Many people who like dairy foods skip them because they think the foods are high in fat. Often, however, this is not the case. Skim milk and low-fat cheeses are not high in fat, but they have just as much calcium as their high-fat counterparts—and often have more. (Table 8.1 identifies many calcium-rich foods.)

In addition to eating calcium-rich foods, people with osteoporosis—or those who are interested in preventing it—may want to include foods containing manganese, a trace metal essential for bone formation. Researcher Jeanne Freeland-Graves, of the University of Texas at Austin, reported at a meeting of the Federation of American Societies for Experimental Biology that levels of manganese in the blood were 33 percent lower in twenty-three women with osteoporosis than in seventeen healthy control subjects. Levels of manganese in the diets of the bone-brittle women were also lower than those of the healthy women.

When the women with osteoporosis ate foods with manganese, they absorbed twice as much of it into the blood as did the other women, suggesting that their bodies have a greater need for the mineral. Some foods that contain manganese are nuts, seeds, pineapples, cereals, beans, and spinach. Of course, this was a rather small study. It's food for thought and for further research—but not necessarily a reason for you to change your diet radically.

There is, however, every reason to increase the amount of calcium-rich foods you consume. In fact, you can add a substantial amount of calcium to your diet and hardly even notice you're doing it. Choose from the many calcium-rich foods listed in Table 8.1 and add more of them to your shopping list. Your body will thank you for it, possibly for decades to come.

9

Hypertension

Millions of Americans regularly eat food without thinking about its sodium content. If they could only have chats with their blood cells and genes, they might be able to hear some sizzling gossip about their eating habits: "You're predisposed to high blood pressure. Stay away—far away—from high-sodium foods or you just might get on the road to developing that life-threatening condition."

But people can't have chats with their systems, so it's often only after too many dill pickles, salted pretzels, bowls of canned, processed soup, or bites of foot-long hot dogs (all high-sodium foods) that they're diagnosed with high blood pressure (also called hypertension), a foot-long, and lifelong, problem.

Research presented at the 1991 meeting of the American Medical Association indicated that unless you are predisposed to developing high blood pressure, you don't have to worry about the sodium content of the food you eat. Many medical experts question that theory. But even if it is true, those same AMA researchers, who unfortunately have given some uninformed dieters a license to shake salt, admit that most people *don't* know they are predisposed to developing high blood pressure until they start showing the symptoms. And the scary thing is that only about 50 percent of people with high blood pressure—a potential killer—are being treated for it.

In fact, the first references to high blood pressure in *How to Control High Blood Pressure Without Drugs,* a widely-hailed book by Dr. Robert L. Rowan of New York University Medical School, call it a "hidden" disease and a "silent killer."

As Dr. Allan Bruckheim writes in his popular syndicated column, "One of the biggest problems with hypertension is that most people don't have any symptoms at all, especially in the early stages. That is why hypertension is called the silent killer."

It is not the hypertension that will actually kill you. It is what the hypertension causes. Hypertension is the most important risk factor for strokes, heart attacks, and kidney failure. As the American Heart Association reports, prolonged high blood pressure also often causes the heart to enlarge, which can lead to arrhythmia (irregularity of the heart's beating) and sudden death.

It is unfortunate that the recent AMA report prompted much-read publications to publish front-page articles with leads like *USA Today*'s: "Don't worry about developing high blood pressure unless it runs in the family, experts now say. . . . About 95 percent of the 60 million people with hypertension have a genetic predisposition."

Those 60 million people represent about one-quarter of the United States population. Other estimates show that one in three people will develop high blood pressure. Several hundred thousand people die each year from diseases related to hypertension. So it's too bad we can't have heart-to-heart chats with our genes.

Other experts discount the genetic predisposition theory regarding hypertension and argue instead that there is a definite link between *anyone's* sodium intake and the development of the disease.

"Hypertension experts gathered . . . to present research that proves a link between sodium intake and high blood pressure for *all* Americans, despite claims that the relationship only affects [the genetically predisposed] minority," the *Los Angeles Times* reported not long before the AMA presented its research.

"Researchers at the Fifth International Interdisciplinary Conference on Hypertension explained that hypertension . . . is a 'populationwide problem.' It is not limited to those who are 'salt-sensitive,' they said, since all Americans are exposed to the same risk factors for hypertension—smoking, obesity, alcohol [abuse], excessive sodium intake, and atherosclerosis," the newspaper reported.

The information from the conference was partially based on a study by Intersalt, a research group that surveyed urine samples of more than 10,000 men and women from thirty-two countries. Intersalt also surveyed the participants, and results from the urine tests and questionnaires found a link between sodium intake and the risk of developing hypertension.

What also makes statements like the AMA's "don't worry about sodium intake" disturbing is that new research indicates that even people with moderate to borderline-high blood pressure are in serious danger of having major health problems.

In the past, it was thought that only those with "high" blood pressure (definition to follow) are at risk for the health problems associated with blood pressure. However, a startling study published in the AMA's own journal reported that about 15 million people with only minimally elevated blood pressure are at risk for developing problems.

"We were surprised to find that individuals with even very minor blood pressure elevation already show signs of damage to their blood vessels and heart," Dr. Stevo Julius, a researcher at the University of Michigan and the principal author of the study, told *People* magazine.

WHAT IS HIGH BLOOD PRESSURE?

Even though so many people develop high blood pressure (or alter their lifestyle or diet to try to prevent the disease), many admit they are not sure exactly what the condition is.

Blood pressure is the force created by the heart as it pushes blood into the arteries and through the circulatory system. As pressure in the arteries rises, the heart must work harder. If the pressure increases above normal, the American Heart Association and other medical groups warn, the result is high blood pressure.

High blood pressure is usually defined as a blood pressure reading of at least 140/90, read as "140 over 90." The first number is the systolic pressure, or the pressure generated as the heart contracts. The bottom number is the diastolic pressure and represents the pressure in the arteries while the heart is filling and resting between beats. High blood pressure is usually diagnosed from at least two separate readings taken on different visits, because mood and stress sometimes temporarily affect readings.

Since there usually are no outward symptoms of high blood pressure, the only way to find out what's happening inside your body is to have your blood pressure checked by a medical professional. This is essential and should be done at least once a year and preferably three or four times. Many pharmacies and public health agencies offer free testing. Children also can have high blood pressure, or levels worth watching, and should be regularly tested once they pass their third birthday.

Beware, however, because even early tests might not predict who will develop problems. A recent study by the University of Southern California showed that many young black women (blacks are at greater risk for the disease) who tested normal later developed health problems related to blood pressure. The USC researchers concluded that preventative diets should be followed by people regardless of what their blood pressure tests reveal.

HOW MUCH SODIUM SHOULD I CONSUME?

Our bodies require only about half a gram of sodium daily, according to the American Heart Association. However, the average American consumes about 6 to 18 grams of salt each day! Food labels often express sodium content in milligrams. The National Academy of Sciences and other health groups advise that to stay in a "safe" range, we should consume 1,100 to 3,300 milligrams (just 0.5 to 1.5 teaspoons) of salt daily. However, those 6 to 18 grams that we actually consume translate into 6,000 to 18,000 milligrams per day!

You might be surprised at just how much sodium many foods have. For example, a serving of one brand's frozen baked lasagna dinner has 1,030 milligrams of sodium; one teaspoon of soy sauce also has 1,030 milligrams; and just one strip of a dill pickle has 430 milligrams.

Look at your food labels. Any ingredient containing the word "salt," "sodium," or "soda" will add sodium to the product. In many products, you may be getting doses of sodium from three or four separate ingredients.

To decrease sodium intake, many experts suggest cooking without salt and then adding it to taste at the table. Switching to unsalted butter or margarine can also be helpful. And lemon juice, lime juice, vinegar, and herbs can all be used as flavorful salt substitutes. Of course, there are many salt substitutes sold commercially, but some of these contain fillers and artificial ingredients that are best avoided. Instead, you may wish to try the herb and spice mixture recommended by the American Heart Association. (See the recipe, below.)

Changing your diet can prevent hypertension, but can it help to lower existing readings? Millions of patients have shown that to be the case. In addition to cutting down on sodium, eating calcium- and potassium-rich foods has been linked with lowering blood pressure. The mineral magnesium, especially, has been shown to help. Some foods containing magnesium are buckwheat

---

All-Natural Salt Substitute

½ teaspoon cayenne pepper
1 tablespoon garlic powder
1 teaspoon dried basil
1 teaspoon dried marjoram
1 teaspoon dried thyme
1 teaspoon dried parsley
1 teaspoon dried savory
1 teaspoon mace
1 teaspoon onion powder
1 teaspoon freshly ground black pepper
1 teaspoon powdered sage

Combine all ingredients, and toss gently with a spoon. Makes about one-third cup. Store in an airtight container in a cool, dry, dark place for up to six months.

pancakes, almonds, bananas, beans, nuts, whole grains, and leafy greens.

"Modifying your eating habits really can work," said Dr. Cleaves Bennett, medical director of the Los Angeles Inner Health Clinic and co-author of *The Control Your High Blood Pressure Cookbook.* "Dietary changes help some people avoid ever having to take blood pressure drugs, and they help others decrease their dosages. And they can work for people who've had blood pressure problems for years."

The best alternative, obviously, is to avoid developing blood pressure problems in the first place. But the good news is that, whatever your blood pressure level is now, changing your diet can make it better. Don't wait until the "silent killer" begins stalking you!

10

Other Ailments

Although not as crippling as cancer, as heartbreaking as heart disease, or as potentially deadly as diabetes, there are plenty of other health, cosmetic, and just downright annoying problems that can occur when one consistently indulges in a poor diet. Let's take a quick look at some of these nutritional "trouble zones."

HEADACHES

The three most frequently experienced types of headaches are migraines, tension headaches, and food-related headaches, according to Dr. Loraine Stern, a clinical professor at the University of California at Los Angeles.

A migraine headache is severe in intensity and is often precipitated by visual disturbances or other physical symptoms. It is experienced as a throbbing, pulsating pain, often concentrated on one side of the head and lasting eight to thirty-six hours. Tension headaches are usually caused by stress. They may involve physical tension of the back or neck muscles.

Food-related headaches start pounding after certain foods are eaten. However, since we tend to eat so many different foods in a given day or week, it is often difficult to distinguish which food might be causing the headache. When someone is under continual stress, what is actually a food-related headache might be mistaken for a tension headache.

To identify a food-related headache, try to pinpoint just when it is you usually get a headache. Is it at work after lunch? Some people chalk up such an occurrence to a stressful day at the office, but it might be worth taking another look to see if a favorite food is usually eaten before the onset of the headache.

One of Stern's patients found out that peanut butter was a culprit in his headaches. Other substances that many people feel are behind their headaches are nitrites (used in the processing of many meats), caffeine, milk, and the additive monosodium glutamate. (Chapters 19 and 20 address caffeine and monosodium glutamate.)

Stern and other physicians suggest keeping a headache diary when it comes to trying to pinpoint a food-related headache. Date, time, severity, and duration of the headache should be noted. What you ate that day and the day before should also be recorded. If the diary (or your own hunch) suggests that certain foods may be involved, cut them from your diet. Then note whether your headaches disappear.

Of course, if you are experiencing constant or very severe headaches, the cause could be something much more serious than certain foods. Stern points out that worrisome signs might include headaches with a sudden onset that become increasingly severe, headaches that awaken you, frequent headaches, and headaches that are not relieved by pain medications. In these instances, you should consult your doctor.

PREMENSTRUAL SYNDROME

More than 70 percent of all women may experience some form of premenstrual syndrome (PMS), according to the Mayo Clinic. Medical journals have been reporting on the syndrome since the 1930s. Although some medical authorities question it as a valid health complaint, Mayo has reported that "a condition this wide-spread demands attention."

Symptoms of PMS typically occur about midway through the menstrual cycle and disappear a few days after a woman finishes her period. Common symptoms include fluid retention, irritability, depression, anxiety, and pain and tenderness of the breasts.

A poor diet can contribute to many of these symptoms. If you eat the kind of nutritionally balanced, natural diet that is advocated throughout this book, you might notice a marked easing of your premenstrual symptoms. Just as important, mounting evidence points to the fact that what you eat and drink prior to and during your menstrual cycle can help prevent many of the symptoms of PMS.

You may want to increase your water consumption. (Regardless of PMS, it's always a good idea to drink eight 8-ounce glasses of water a day.) Drinking lots of water can help flush out your system and therefore help prevent fluid retention. Another good way to reduce fluid retention is to eat less salt and salty foods prior to and during your period.

When it comes to other types of food, it might be better to increase rather than limit your consumption of them. "Relief from premenstrual syndrome may lie only a potato salad away. Researchers at the Massachusetts Institute of Technology have found that eating carbohydrates often relieves the emotional symptoms of depression, anger, and anxiety that accompany PMS," the nutrition letter of *Eating Well* magazine reported.

Other studies have shown that high-carbohydrate foods increase brain levels of serotonin, a substance known to induce calmness. Potatoes and whole-grain pasta are high-carbohydrate foods that are recommended as good dietary choices before and during the menstrual cycle.

Judith Wurtman, the cell biologist who conducted the MIT study, has said women should not deny themselves indulgences in high-carbohydrate foods before and during their menstrual cycle. "In essence, eating high-carbohydrate foods is a way for PMS women to medicate themselves," she told *Eating Well* magazine. "It may not be as powerful as a drug, but it also does not have as many side effects."

The following dietary tips from the Mayo Clinic may help ease PMS symptoms:

- Don't drink alcohol a few days prior to your menstrual period.
- Avoid products that contain caffeine, such as coffee, tea, and

cola-based soft drinks, just before and during your period. This may help reduce tension and irritability.

- As the MIT study pointed out, eat more complex carbohydrates. In addition to potatoes, this can include bread, rice, cereal, and vegetables. Try to avoid, however, simple sugars, such as table sugar, honey, sugar-sweetened soda, and candy.

- Limit fatty cuts of meat and cold cuts, butter, margarine, whole milk, and ice cream.

- Substitute smaller, more frequent meals for three large meals. Don't skip meals.

- Although vitamin B$_6$ is sometimes recommended for PMS, the Mayo Clinic advises against taking more than 500 milligrams a day. Nerve damage is a possible risk when large doses of the vitamin are consumed.

SLEEP DISORDERS

Researchers estimate that the average number of hours you will sleep in your lifetime is 220,000. What you regularly eat, however, could lop off more than a few hours from that lifetime average. On the other hand, sleep-promoting foods may help you accumulate lots of hours of peaceful sleep.

Doctors use the term "parasomnias" to refer to conditions that interfere with normal sleep. These conditions can range from slight disturbances to those that seriously affect one's ability to sleep. Certain ingredients in foods can be parasomnias or can aggravate existing parasomnias.

Caffeine—a drug that's a stimulant—is chief among the substances in food that can aggravate sleep. To ensure that caffeine does not affect your ability to fall asleep, try and avoid it from the early afternoon on—if not completely.

Until they cut down or cut out their use of caffeine, some people don't even realize that it is affecting their ability to sleep. Rose Jollop, a Southern California senior citizen, thought she was a night owl. She wouldn't begin to feel drowsy until 12:30 or 1:00 a.m. She would then wake up in the late morning and not feel completely rested. After reading a lot about caffeine a few years ago, Jollop decided to cut it from her diet. To her surprise, she found she would begin to feel drowsy at 10:00 or 10:30 p.m. and wake up—feeling much more rested than when she had used caffeine—at 7:00 a.m.

Alcohol makes some people drowsy. Actually, though, this is deceiving. Much research proves that although alcohol may initially make a person sleepy, during the sleep cycle it causes disturbances. Also, of course, no one would want to grow dependent on alcohol as a sleep aid.

"Alcohol is one of the least effective sleep medications on the open market," wrote a team of Harvard University doctors in *Your Good Health: How to Stay Well*, a book published by Harvard University.

"Although it usually induces drowsiness, within hours after an alcoholic drink is taken a kind of withdrawal syndrome develops and disrupts sleep," they continued. "What begins as a kind of dopey slumber easily turns into a night of tossing and turning. . . . People who have difficulty sleeping are well advised to minimize their alcohol intake in general and to drink nothing after the dinner hour."

The consumption of spicy foods also can influence sleep. Try not to eat such foods late in the evening. Also, as most people know, it's best to stay away from very large meals in the evening. As your body tries to digest such a feast, you may toss and turn or find it difficult to fall asleep. However, if you find that you have awakened in the night and you feel hungry, it's best to go ahead and have a light snack.

While some foods and beverages can play havoc with your ability to sleep, others are clearly your friends. You may have heard of tryptophan. Some of the tablet forms of tryptophan, an essential amino acid, came under scrutiny a few years ago because they were packed unsanitarily. However, tryptophan occurs naturally in many foods and can help nudge you into drowsiness.

Tryptophan is found in turkey, bananas, and dairy products. If you eat a food containing tryptophan to help induce sleep, it is wise also to eat a carbohydrate (like a whole-grain cracker) with it. The carbohydrate can increase the sleep-promoting effects of tryptophan, which when it enters the brain helps to form serotonin, a substance that helps bring on sleep.

And if you reach for a dairy product like milk, it is indeed best to warm it up. Warm milk really can help promote sleep. The heat makes the calcium—a natural sedative—more available to the body. Insomnia prevention is just another reason to be sure you regularly eat a calcium-rich diet.

Research has also shown that vitamin B_1—thiamine—helps conquer sleep disturbances. Thiamine is a part of the vitamin B complex found in such foods as beans, egg yolks, and liver.

Many people have found certain herbs helpful when it comes to promoting sleep. The five herbs usually recommended for those who would like a gentle boost into dreamland are blue vervain, catnip, hops, valerian, and passion flower. These are all available as teas. Herb experts also recommend adding a bit of milk (for its tryptophan and calcium) to such a tea.

FOOD ALLERGIES AND SENSITIVITIES

Allergies trigger the body's immune system. If allergies go untreated, they can seriously weaken that system. Symptoms of food allergies can be immediate or can manifest themselves hours after eating. Symptoms include headaches, vomiting, stomach cramps, diarrhea, and hives. Some of the most common culprits behind food allergies are milk products, corn, eggs, wheat, sugar, coffee, nuts, chocolate, coconut, artificial additives, citrus, pork, fish, soy, and potatoes.

Any substance to which your body is allergic is called an allergen. Once your body learns it is allergic to something, it makes proteins called antibodies to fight the allergens. Whenever it is exposed to the allergen again—even in a small dosage—it will fight it. Some allergies can be fatal.

Food sensitivities (also called intolerances) are far more common than food allergies and generally don't produce as harsh a reaction. They also don't call into play the body's immune system. One of the most common food sensitivities is lactose intolerance, which is the inability to digest milk products.

Many people suffer from food sensitivities without realizing it. They may crave the very foods that are playing havoc with their systems. For example, many people are sensitive to refined sugar.

They might not realize, though, that their mood swings, skin break-outs, and weight gains are due to their sensitivity to sugar, and they may crave the food more than any other. Only by cutting the food out of their diet would they realize the effect it was having upon them.

When you're truly allergic to a food, you should avoid eating it. However, if you are merely sensitive to a food, it may be because you are not eating a big enough variety of foods. If you eat only a small number of foods, you can develop a sensitivity to one or more of them, according to Dr. Harvey Ross, a Los Angeles nutritionist who has written a number of books on food sensitivity. Relying on an additive-filled diet—or chronically undernourishing yourself by relying mainly on junk foods—can also be behind many food sensitivities.

If you want to determine if you might be sensitive to a given food, Dr. Ross suggests that you don't eat the suspected food for four days. If symptoms lessen, eat the suspected food by itself on an empty stomach (at least two hours after eating). If the symptoms recur, the food is probably a trigger for food sensitivities. You then may want to avoid the food.

If you want to determine if you're allergic to a given food, you might need an allergist to diagnose the problem.

COSMETIC PROBLEMS

If you don't like the condition of your hair, skin, or nails, it might be wiser to take a look at your diet instead of at the products on the shelves of your local beauty supply shop. In fact, some of the miracle "cures" promised by some beauty products can be achieved much more quickly by eating a nutritious diet.

For example, let's say you have very thin hair or even some balding. While, of course, this could be a result of your family tree, it can also be a result of a poor diet. Some hair follicles are always dormant. But having too many hair follicles dormant at once can result in thin hair or balding.

Dormant hair follicles can be the result of a poor diet. Low-protein diets, crash diets, and diets that severely restrict calories have been known to cause such problems. The good news is that once good nutrition replaces poor nutrition, hair follicles most likely will gradually become active again and sprout new hair.

If your diet is fairly good but it lacks food rich in the mineral zinc, you will probably experience hair and skin problems. In a 1989 study reported in the *Journal of Applied Nutrition*, patients with a severe form of acne had almost 30 percent less zinc in their blood and about 25 percent less zinc in their hair than those without acne.

Hair or skin problems involving zinc as a culprit are caused by having too little of that mineral in the diet. However, when it comes to skin problems involving iodine in the diet, it's a different story. A recent study showed that people who ate foods containing a lot of iodine were more likely to experience acne flare-ups.

Fast-food meals have a high iodine content that can aggravate acne, according to Dr. Harvey Arbesman, a dermatologist at the State University of New York at Buffalo. His analysis found that a burger-and-French-fries meal in a fast-food restaurant can contain up to thirty times the daily requirement of iodine. Arbesman wrote about his findings in a 1990 edition of the *New England Journal of Medicine*, where he also reiterated the well-known fact that even small amounts of excess iodine can cause acne eruptions.

Even with all the advertising out there having to do with hair and skin products, a nutritious diet is probably the best available beauty regimen. "A good balance of protein, fats, and carbohydrates, with adequate amounts of vitamins and minerals, is essential for skin health," according to Gilbert Martin of the American Academy of Dermatology. "Maintaining a well-balanced healthful diet will provide your body with all the nutrients you need to have healthy hair, skin, and nails."

Maintaining such a diet may, of course, be easier said than done, especially with all of the confusing and often contradictory information blaring at us consumers every day. In Part II, we'll take a close-up, specific look at many of the hot nutritional topics of the day, and learn how we can get the most nutrition out of every bite we take.

Part II
How You Can Eat Better: Exploring the Issues

11

Water

If you had told Phoenix's Sue Jergenson ten years ago that she'd be rushing through her busy day with a 51-ounce bottle of expensive water tucked under her arm, or that she'd be keeping a twelve-dollar stock of such bottles in her office refrigerator, or that she would be running out in the wee hours of the morning for replacement bottles, she would have said you were crazy.

"Ten years ago, it would have been cigarettes that I had stockpiled in my desk or was running out in the evening to buy," said Jergenson, a stockbroker and former smoker.

However, Jergenson is an avid consumer of one of the largest and fastest-growing bottled beverage industries in the world: the water industry.

But as many of us swig our bottled water or run to our tap to refill our cups—and swallow the eight glasses a day we may have heard are essential for weight loss and good health—nearly as many of us are unsure about the quality of the water we drink or about the true health benefits of keeping our body's "water tank" full. Read on, and we'll take a look at those issues until they are as crystal clear and sparkling as a tall glass of H_2O.

WATER: WHAT'S ALL THE FUSS ABOUT?

Did you know that your body is one-half to two-thirds water? That means if you weigh 150 pounds, 90 pounds of that may be water.

There are just six classes of nutrients: Carbohydrates, fat, protein, vitamins, minerals, and water. Although most people can go for months without most of the other elements, water needs to be replenished within a few days or you can become seriously ill or even die.

Close to 50 percent of your body's water weight is inside your cells. About 20 percent surrounds the cells, and the rest is in your blood vessels.

Many of us have heard that for good health we should try to drink eight 8-ounce glasses of water per day. Medical experts recommend that amount because that is just about how much water the average person loses through sweat, urine, and other sources each day. If you exercise a lot or are active in hot weather, you should drink even more than eight glasses a day.

It is essential to replenish your body's water supply. The water in your body transports nutrients and wastes, ensures proper chemical reactions, cushions and lubricates the joints, regulates your temperature, and softens the skin. Without enough water, kidneys do not function properly.

It's true that drinking plenty of water can help you lose weight. This has to do with the liver's taking over for the kidneys if you are not drinking enough water. Part of the liver's function is to metabolize fat into energy. However, when the liver is substituting for the kidneys, it is less efficient at burning fat. In that case, weight loss can slow down.

Therefore, when you drink more water, you can burn more fat. Because drinking water can also flush out your system, you will be less likely to retain water—and retained water puffs up both you and the number you see on your scale. Those watching their weight should try to drink eight 8-ounce glasses of water per day. Add an extra glass for every twenty-five pounds of excess weight.

What about other foods and beverages? Can't you get plenty of water into your system by eating or drinking those? In fact, many foods are mostly water. Most fruits are more than 80 percent water, while vegetables range from 70 to 95 percent. Eggs are 75 percent water, meat can be 40 to 80 percent water, and most breads are about 30 percent water. You do receive water from those sources, but it is still important to try to drink about eight glasses of water a day.

Relying on sugar-filled or caffeinated beverages for part of your water intake is not a good idea. These beverages do not move through your body as cleanly as does water. Sugar in beverages, for example, can, according to the Mayo Clinic, keep fluid in your stomach for a longer time. Caffeine-containing beverages, as well as having the pharmaceutical and other effects described in Chapter 19, act as diuretics, which take away from your fluid level rather than adding to it. Even decaffeinated coffee or tea contains chemicals that act as diuretics.

Infants and toddlers shouldn't be left out of the water revolution. A baby has a higher risk of dehydration than an adult has because there is a greater proportion of water in his or her tiny body. Water can also help promote waste elimination and help an infant's barely-formed kidneys do their job. Consult a pediatrician to find out how much water your infant or child should be drinking.

Is it possible to drink too much water? In most cases, the answer is no, but there are some rare cases where a type of addiction or intoxication has occurred.

Marathoners on occasion have taken in too much water without replacing the salt lost from their bodies. This intoxication has caused convulsions and comas. To avoid such a situation, a cup of fluid should not be drunk more than every 15 minutes if you are exercising in the heat. If you are exercising for a long period, something containing salt should also be eaten or drunk.

A rare psychiatric condition can cause people to become compulsive water drinkers. Such people consume up to three gallons of water a day, which can cause severe brain damage, seizures, vomiting, coma, or death.

However, the average person who has drunk too much water might merely feel bloated or slightly nauseated.

If you are on a severely salt-restricted diet, you might need to take into consideration the kind of water you are drinking. The average amount of sodium in public tap water in the United States is about 47 milligrams per quart; but, according to the Mayo

Clinic, softened water can be double that. Water is softened by removing calcium and magnesium and adding sodium. This is known as an ion exchange process.

"If you need to control sodium, and your water contains more than 40 milligrams of sodium per quart (ask the softening company), use distilled or purified water (they have had salt removed) for drinking or cooking. Or simply be sure that your cold tap is not connected to the softener, and use that tap for drinking and cooking," wrote the editors of the *Mayo Clinic Nutrition Letter* in a recent advisory.

QUALITY CONCERNS

Be forewarned: Don't let the following information stop you from drinking water.

Although some quality concerns exist, the benefits of drinking water are real. That's why it is important to make an informed choice by learning as much as we can about the water we drink. If you have questions about drinking water, you can have it analyzed. To find out how, or for any other water information, call the Environmental Protection Agency's (EPA's) Safe Drinking Water Hotline at (800) 426–4791; from Washington D.C. or Alaska, call (202) 382–5533.

Many of us have seen a lot of the negative publicity tap water has received in recent years. Unfortunately, there are many areas of concern.

According to the United States Centers for Disease Control (CDC), an average of about 7,500 cases of illness related to drinking water were reported in the United States each year from 1970 to 1985. The CDC has stated that the number of reported cases reflects only a fraction of the cases that actually occur.

Contamination can occur even though about 80 percent of the nation's drinking water supply is protected by the EPA's Safe Drinking Water Act, which sets limits on certain contaminants in water. The EPA, however, has set limits for about only fifty contaminants. They are directed by law to regulate another twenty-five within each three-year period until they feel they have regulated all existing contaminants. Why, however, should bureaucracy and the slow wheels of government be affecting the quality of our water? How is this helpful to us as we swallow that water? It is a shame more people can't work more hours to regulate all contaminants now rather than bureaucratically look at only a certain number every three years.

What are some of the contaminants that can be in drinking water? They include microorganisms (such as bacteria and viruses), nitrates from fertilizer or sewage, and lead that can seep into water from lead pipes in your home. If your home was built or remodeled before 1985—prior to the ban on lead pipes—it may harbor levels of excess lead.

Almost 60 percent of Americans use public water systems whose source is the surface water from reservoirs, lakes, or rivers. The other 40 percent of the population use ground-water sources. Unfortunately, during the last twenty years, new chemicals have been among the contaminants to invade both ground and surface water outlets. Water invaders can include pesticide and fertilizer runoff from farmland, industrial wastes, leaking underground storage tanks, and septic tank discharge.

Because of pesticide runoffs, many water experts are fans of organic farming (which we'll go over in Chapter 21). Arthur Saarinen, president of the Water Pollution Control Federation—which in 1990 hosted a pollution control conference attended by 13,000 water experts from around the world—said at a press conference that organic farming is definitely important to the safety of the water supply.

IS BOTTLED BETTER?

Because many people and businesses have concerns about their tap water, the bottled water business is booming. It is the fastest growing segment of the beverage industry. During the last ten years, sales have surged by 500 percent. It is a $2.5 billion industry.

However, there are also questions about the quality of bottled water. Many sources where the water is bottled are not regulated. Also, some bottled waters may just be bottled tap water. Even if your bottled water isn't bottled tap water, it can have contamination problems.

Researchers from Northeastern University recently discovered some startling facts when they sampled eight different bottled brands. They discovered in the water several types of bacteria, often the same kind that has been found in tap water.

However, tap water runs, the researchers pointed out, but bottled water lies dormant for extended periods. "The number of bacteria increases with storage, since the organisms can attach to the sides and bottom of the [inside of the] container and rapidly multiply," said microbiologist Fred Rosenberg, who was on the study team. For most healthy people, bacteria like those present in bottled waters present no extreme danger but can cause intestinal problems like diarrhea, Rosenberg said.

Further Northeastern University studies on bottled water turned up more bacteria. The researchers also pointed out that although water may show no bacteria at a packaging plant, it almost always shows some when it reaches a consumer's home. Refrigeration can help cut bacteria in bottled water. If you want to be on the ultra-safe side, then follow Rosenberg's suggestion to boil the water for three or more minutes after removing it from the bottle. That kills all the bacteria.

WATER WISDOM

I repeat: Don't let concern about contamination stop you from drinking water. And there are a number of things you can do to make sure the water you drink is safe and healthful. First, if you use a public water supply, contact your local utility and request a copy of any water analysis they have performed; if you drink bottled water, contact the company for this information. If your water comes from another source, such as a private well, you can obtain a testing kit from a certified independent laboratory (preferably one that is not also in the water treatment business) that can test samples and provide you with an analysis of your water.

If you determine that your water contains unacceptable levels of chemicals, bacteria, or other pollutants, and you are unable to switch to a healthier water source, you might want to consider using some type of filtration system. An increasingly popular option is the so-called point-of-source filter system, which attaches to a single faucet in your home. There are several different kinds available, including carbon block, reverse osmosis, combination carbon block/reverse osmosis, and distiller units. They operate in different ways, and prices vary. All remove bacteria and other microorganisms, but their effectiveness against other pollutants varies. Before investing in any filter unit, make sure that it will work on the problem substances that you want removed from your water.

If you are worried about the possibility of excess lead in your water, one precaution you can take is to let the water run for a few minutes before using it. That way, lead that may have leached into the water from plumbing pipes will be largely flushed out.

Whether you choose to take it from the tap or the bottle, it is important to know as much as you can about the water you drink. The main thing to remember, though, is that you simply can't live without water.

12

Sugars and Sweeteners

A product label that says "no refined sugar" can mislead a consumer into thinking he or she is getting a sugar-free product. The product may have no refined sugar, but it often may contain processed sugars, like high-fructose corn syrup (which is the result of a manufacturing process we'll describe shortly). Also, products list their ingredients by descending order according to weight, but this system can be misleading when it comes to sugar and some other ingredients.

A manufacturer may list one ingredient as sugar, another as high-fructose corn syrup, a third as brown sugar or molasses, and distribute them throughout the ingredients list. But if all sugars were listed together (as the Center for Science in the Public Interest has suggested), sugar would then be listed as the product's primary ingredient.

There are differences between the sugars in our foods. Aficionados of "whole" foods would recommend looking for foods sweetened with fruit juice, honey, or fructose (fruit sugar). Those choices are in their natural, more nutrient-dense state and are unrefined. Rice syrup is also a natural sweetener.

Some food manufacturers will tell you that all sugars (refined fructose, honey, and the like) are alike. All sugars are basically digested alike—quickly, which is why they translate to quick energy (although sugar from fruit and honey are digested a bit more slowly). However, much of the similarity ends there.

Lots of manufacturers put large lettering on their packages claiming "all natural." A close look at the ingredients, however, shows that some of those products are mainly refined sugar. The chemical formula for sugar is $C_{12}H_{22}O_{11}$. Multiple chemical processing of the sugar cane or sugar beet (the natural substances the manufacturers are referring to) produces sugar. That process, however, removes all fiber and protein, both of which made up 90 percent of the original sugar plant. This is truly what is meant by "empty calories," the term frequently applied to substances like refined sugar, which has 2,500 calories per pound. And yet refined sugar is by far the top additive in packaged foods today, with the average person consuming 130 pounds of it a year.

What's the difference between sugar and honey? William Dufty explains the facts well in *Sugar Blues*, a best-seller hailed by consumers and medical experts:

"Pure is a favorite adjective of the sugar pushers because it means one thing to chemists and another thing to the ordinary mortals. When honey is labeled pure, this means that it is in its natural state (stolen directly from the bees who made it), no adulteration with sucrose to stretch it and no harmful chemical residues which men have sprayed on the flowers. It does not mean the honey is free from (beneficial) minerals like iodine, iron, calcium, phosphorous, or multiple vitamins. So effective is the purification process which sugar cane and beets undergo in the refineries, that sugar ends up as chemically pure as the morphine and heroin a chemist has on his laboratory shelves. What nutritional virtue this abstract chemical purity represents, the sugar pushers never tell us."

If you are a reader of food product labels, you have probably noticed a lot of listings for high-fructose corn syrup. This is not the same thing as fructose, which is unadulterated fruit sugar.

High-fructose corn syrup is used as a cheap substitute for refined sugar. Almost all soft drinks and many other packaged food products use it. According to the Mayo Clinic's report on high-fructose corn syrup in its *Nutrition Letter*, the additive gained wide acceptance when sugar prices rose between 1974 and 1980.

High-fructose corn syrup now makes up half of all sugar consumption, according to Mayo.

High-fructose corn syrup contains fructose, while regular corn syrup, also used as a sweetener, does not. High-fructose corn syrup is made from corn by food companies that chemically change glucose in cornstarch to fructose. Quite a difference from a product that is sweetened by, say, 100-percent grape juice!

SACCHARIN AND ASPARTAME

What about other sweetening choices? Many of us now stay away from the additive saccharin. Studies showed that it caused cancer in some laboratory animals, and every product that contains it now sports a health warning on its label. That is certainly enough to keep most health-conscious people from reaching for saccharin-filled products.

Perhaps it should also be a lesson about what happens when human beings take over a job that has always been performed by nature. Prior to saccharin, all sweeteners were natural. Saccharin, the first man-made sugar substitute, is 300 to 400 times sweeter than sugar.

Although saccharin use has dwindled since the publicity about its links to cancer, we now have thousands of products—and the list is always growing—that are sweetened instead with low-calorie aspartame (marketed under the brand names Equal and NutraSweet). In its many print and television ads, NutraSweet boasts how natural it is. Let's take a closer look.

Aspartame is an example of the kind of foods many scientists are concocting for us in laboratories. It went through more than a hundred tests over eight years before it was approved. However, many health groups still question the safety of chemically, scientifically derived products like aspartame. (We'll look at the results of some of the aspartame tests in a moment.)

Aspartame was only introduced into the marketplace in 1981, so there is no way to know its possible long-term effects. The FDA seconds that opinion, since it will never grant permanent approval to any additive but rather keeps the door open for further testing. However, just because further testing might be needed, that doesn't stop such ingredients from infiltrating the food supply.

NutraSweet has boasted to us in its television spots that from its modest beginnings in one single gum ball it is now in more than 4,000 products. Other information about aspartame shows, in fact, that it is the world's number one selling sugar substitute. Scientists are feverishly working to get NutraSweet into every possible product, eventually to replace sugar completely, the company's chairman says.

Commercials for NutraSweet tell us it is made up of amino acids—compounds of protein—just like a banana or other food. However, aspartame was actually discovered accidentally by a scientist at a pharmaceutical company who was developing an ulcer drug. It is a methyl ester of the peptides phenylalanine and aspartic acid and, therefore, is metabolized as a protein. It is painstakingly manufactured in a lab by chemists in white coats using long computer-automated robot arms. Very little resemblance to a banana or any other natural food!

Even though the list of aspartame-containing products grows almost daily, there are notations in the scientific literature about its safety—warnings we have never seen on any product label in the supermarket. The *Journal of the American Dietetic Association* states, "Based on long-term testing, moderate consumption of the sweetener has been shown to be safe." To me, the following ADA statement, which defines "moderate consumption" of aspartame, is a shocker. The ADA states that "moderate, safe levels of NutraSweet for a 130-pound person have been determined at 18 packets of NutraSweet, or three cans of diet soda a day."

Many people drink more than three cans of diet soda per day. Most of them, I'm sure, are completely unaware of this ADA directive, which has been verified by other nutrition experts as well. Plus, that measure for "moderate" consumption does not apply to everyone. What if you weigh less than 130 pounds—as many women who drink lots of diet soda do?

The first article I wrote as a health reporter was for an international press syndicate and brought out the fact that the high acid level of diet soda can damage the teeth. I talked to many average people who drink six cans of diet soda per day! Also, with aspartame in so many other products (hot chocolate, juice drinks, frozen yogurt, gelatin, breath mints, sugar-free gum), it would be quite easy for someone drinking three cans of diet soda a day to be ingesting much more aspartame than just what is in the soda.

The uproar over saccharin involved tests that showed it would be possibly damaging if someone consumed 850 or more cans of diet soda in one day. Yet, with products containing aspartame, which carry no general warning, the amount recommended by the ADA for safety is only three cans of diet soda a day!

What are the possible health worries when it comes to aspartame? Aspartame is a methyl ester of two amino acids: L-aspartic acid and L-phenylalanine. The *Journal of the American Dietetic Association* reported that elevated levels of phenylalanine "have the potential to induce brain lesions." The ADA states that this would *probably* take much higher doses of aspartame than what the average person would consume.

The journal immediately followed the statement about possible brain lesions and high doses of aspartame with this (all emphases mine): "Aspartame, along with carbohydrates, increases cerebral levels of the branch-chain amino acids, as well as phenylalanine and tyrosine. Branch-chain amino acids compete with phenylalanine and tyrosine for transport across the blood-brain barrier. Ingestion of aspartame with carbohydrate appears to potentiate this competition and results in a decrease in the levels of serotonin, which normally increase after a carbohydrate meal.

"*The clinical significance of this is unknown.* While aspartame is *probably* safe in this regard *at low consumption levels*, the question of the relationship of aspartame to neurobiochemical effects in human beings *requires additional research.* In 1983, the FDA stated that it is *reasonably* certain that aspartame does not cause brain tumors, brain damage or behavioral changes. Another issue is the possibility that aspartame, either alone or in combination with glutamate, may contribute to brain damage, resulting in mental retardation or adversely affecting the neuroendocrine regulatory system."

The *Journal of the American Dietetic Association* also notes the investigation of less serious health problems that are possibly due to aspartame. The Center for Science in the Public Interest has investigated more than 500 reports of symptoms that users felt were due to their intake of the sweetener. Symptoms included stomach upsets, hives, headaches, menstrual problems, insomnia, and uncontrolled behavior.

Why don't more people just enjoy natural sweeteners like honey or fructose or fruit juice rather than wait years for the results of elaborate scientific tests on man-made sweeteners to determine whether they may be playing Russian roulette with their health? As much as the ADA is an important organization that lets the public know about much essential health information, I think the conclusion they draw at the end of their *Journal of the American Dietetic Association* article "Position of the ADA: Appropriate Use of Nutritive and Non-Nutritive Sweeteners" is a scary one. It shows that they—and other mainstream nutrition organizations like them—often shoot for the lowest common denominator when it comes to their faith in our being able to eat for vitality.

Instead of urging a person to eat natural sweeteners for health (where no scientific tests or questions about brain lesions or bladder cancer are necessary), they sum up their report on aspartame, saccharin, and even cyclamate (which we'll describe in a moment) by stating, "An individual can minimize potential risks from any one sweetener by using a variety of available sweeteners, thus ingesting less of any specific sweetener. Research into possible risks of long-term use of non-nutritive sweeteners, either alone or in combinations, should continue."

My question is, when there are natural alternatives readily available (which have been shown to help with weight loss even more than human-created sweeteners, as we'll discuss in a moment), why pass them up to become a guinea pig for ongoing experiments regarding the artificial sweeteners?

THE RECALL OF SWEETENERS

Aspartame might of course, never be pulled from our food supply. But other sweeteners people exposed themselves to for years have been banned, proving that we as individuals must be aware of data surrounding a new additive rather than wait decades to be told we may have been contaminating ourselves.

Cyclamate, a sugar substitute widely used through 1970, was shown to be a possible cause of bladder cancer and was eventually banned from products. But, as Michael Jacobson, Ph.D., director of the Center for Science in the Public Interest, reported, even fifteen years later the company that sold cyclamate was still asking the FDA to allow its use. The *Los Angeles Times* reported in 1990 that cyclamate manufacturers were still petitioning the FDA.

Xylitol, another sugar substitute touted as a great way to avoid tooth decay, was used in Care Free gum, Life Savers, and other products in the 1970s. It originated in Finland and was approved for use by the FDA in 1963, but studies later found that it seemed to promote bladder tumors in laboratory animals. American companies stopped using xylitol. According to the Center for Science in the Public Interest, an FDA official said: "It had to be conceded that xylitol appeared to induce tumors in a dose-related manner in both rats and mice." Although the FDA proposed banning xylitol, it never completed the action. Today some candies imported into the United States from Finland still contain the additive.

SUGAR AND LOW-CALORIE SWEETENERS AS POSSIBLE SABOTEURS TO WEIGHT LOSS

Even people who regularly choose products containing aspartame or other low-calorie sweeteners precisely so they will lose weight may not realize just how much high-calorie refined sugar they are still eating along with their "diet" products.

When frequent dieters, for example, pop a Lean Cuisine frozen lasagna into their oven, most are probably not even considering the fact that sugars would be a player in a food used for weight control. But in addition to many other ingredients, sugar makes an appearance three separate times in this entrée: Sugar is added to the overall product, it is an ingredient in the "mushroom base," and it is added in the form of sugar-cane syrup.

Because I am a food editor at a daily newspaper, I was sent a sample of Basic 4, a new cereal from General Mills that brags about how nutritious it is because it includes ingredients from every food group. With notices like that on the front of the cereal box, many shoppers might just pop it into their shopping carts without reading the tiny ingredients list on the side panel.

Incredibly, though, there are six different sugars staggered throughout that list, and that doesn't even count the four different fruits that are also in the product. The sugars are sugar, brown sugar, fructose, corn syrup, sorbitol (a sugar substitute), and brown sugar syrup. The cereal has questionable preservatives and artificial flavor. The fruits that add to the powerful sweetness (and overall sugar count) of this cereal are raisins, cranberries, dried apples, and prune juice concentrate.

The sugar substitute sorbitol is an example of just how much some of these sweeteners mixed for us in packaged foods actually get around. It is a sweet, crystalline alcohol obtained from the berries of the mountain ash. Proving its versatility, it is also suitable for use as a moistening agent in lotions and creams! Many companies (General Mills on its Basic 4 cereal package *not* being one of them) warn on their labels that sorbitol may also moisten your insides, causing—as it does in many people when they eat dietetic sorbitol-sweetened candy—immediate diarrhea.

As much as diet products like Lean Cuisine or those sweetened with aspartame or sorbitol tout themselves, there has never been any conclusive proof that calorie-reduced products are actually helpful when it comes to losing weight. According to a 1989 report by the Institute of Food Technologists' Expert Panel on Food Safety and Nutrition, "Low-calorie food and ingredients (including sweeteners) cannot offer quick fixes or serve as magic bullets to weight loss or control." It went on to say, "So far there is no evidence that the proliferation of these foods have had any effect on how fat Americans are." In fact, although 80 million Americans —about one in three—say they follow weight-control diets and use low-calorie sweeteners, obesity is still increasing rapidly rather than going down.

Of course, if you ate only low-calorie foods you would lose weight. But, study after study has shown that just because we are eating lots of the new low-calorie products, we are not necessarily eating less of the high-calorie foods. Therefore, we still gain weight. Also, the acclaimed Monnell Chemistry and Research Center in Philadelphia has shown, and other organizations' studies have verified, that in low-calorie products certain ingredients—especially aspartame—may actually cause our brain to tell us we are hungrier and not satiated.

Another study on artificial sweeteners also did not offer good news for dieters. The data on weight changes in 78,694 women who were involved in an American Cancer Society mortality study from 1968 to 1988 showed that women who used artificial sweeteners were actually more likely to gain weight than those who did not.

However, when you eat something sweetened naturally, studies have shown, it is possible to lose weight without even trying and without slaving away at non-existent weight loss.

A 1988 Yale University study had twenty-four women and men between ages twenty-two and fifty drink lemonade sweetened with either fructose (natural fruit sugar) or refined sugar. About thirty minutes later, the subjects were offered a buffet lunch. Those who had drunk the fructose beverage consumed an average of 30 percent fewer calories and chose less fatty foods than the other test participants. The researchers recommended from their study that those trying to lose weight consume a piece of fruit or a glass of 100-percent fruit juice as an appetizer prior to their meals.

SWEETENERS: WHAT THE FUTURE HOLDS

Plenty of artificial sweeteners have just hit the market or are being tested for future use. However, as we've seen, even many sweeteners (as well as other foods) that have been tested and end up on our supermarket shelves are deemed to raise serious health questions and require further testing—presumably as we spoon them each day into our morning coffee or breakfast cereals.

In 1991, Canada became the first country to try diet foods and beverages sweetened with sucralose, a new low-calorie sweetener marketed under the name Splenda. A petition for its use in the United States is pending before the FDA. There are also petitions for ten other sweeteners.

Another sugar substitute, unnamed but in development since 1990, is a combination of sorbitol and mannitol. Mannitol is a sweetener like sorbitol that is also used as a dusting or anti-sticking agent in food products. According to the *Consumer's Dictionary of Food Additives*, "in excess (like sorbitol) it can cause gastrointestinal disturbances. It may also induce or worsen kidney disease."

Acesulfame-K was approved for United States use in 1990. Its brand name is Sunette, and it is being marketed to consumers as Sweet One. It is a man-made sweetener that is 200 times sweeter than sugar. It was tested for six years and has been used in Europe since 1986.

The Center for Science in the Public Interest, however, has filed a formal objection asking the FDA to withdraw its approval of the sweetener. They question the FDA's approval because the results of one of the rat studies done on acesulfame-K showed about double the amount of mammary gland tumors in the group of rats fed Sunette compared with the control group. However, the FDA decision was based on the fact that that strain of rat shows a somewhat higher incidence of breast tumors in general. I'd add my voice to that of the Center for Science in the Public Interest and ask, why was such a group of rats used? And why wouldn't another set of tests with different strains of rats be done—just in case?

I'm not the only one who should be thinking up additional questions. Whether it's Sunette or sucralose or any new sweetener that comes down the pike in years to come, why not ask yourself: Why was this sweetener developed? Is it because it's a great, healthful product for me to enjoy?

Often, those are not the reasons food products are developed. The artificial sweetener industry, according to recent figures compiled by the *Los Angeles Times*, generates one billion dollars annually. The decision to create sweeteners is usually directly related to how the industry can further increase that figure.

The sorbitol-and-mannitol sweetener mixture, for example, was created, according to the Institute of Food Technologists, because the combination creates less of an aftertaste than many other "fake" sugars. (Natural sweeteners don't leave any aftertaste.) Sucralose was developed because it can last longer than its competitors in food products and still stay sweet. Acesulfame-K is "highly regarded by food technologists" because it can be used for baking and high-heat cooking, wrote Daniel Puzo, investigative food writer for the *Los Angeles Times*. "Nutrasweet has been limited in its food applications because it does not break down when exposed to the high temperatures required for baking or stove-top cooking."

Many of these sweeteners (sucralose and the mannitol blend, for example) are created mainly for combined use with other man-made sweeteners like NutraSweet and saccharin. As the ADA, the Center for Science in the Public Interest, and many other nutrition researchers point out, however, even if tests on individual man-made sweeteners have shown marginal safety zones, they have not been tested in combination with other sweeteners. There is no way to know what the potential health effect of combined sweeteners might be.

Few people would willingly eliminate the pleasure of eating sweet treats from their lives altogether, and I'm not really suggesting that we should. But in light of all the things we don't know about the effects of artificial sweeteners—and all the things we do know about the effects of refined sugar—it makes sense for health-concerned people to choose foods that use natural sweeteners. You can pass up both the empty calories of refined sugar and the questionable concoctions of food-company laboratories, and still wake up to that sweet cup of tea or bowl of cereal.

13

Fats and Oils

Sheila Everson never thought she would be intrigued by olive oil. Yet the Nashville housewife has invested a small fortune in learning about the bottle of liquid that now regularly occupies a spot in her kitchen pantry. She bought a cookbook of recipes that use olive oil, and she took a class at her local community center on the virtues of cooking with the oil. Why the fuss? Everson, like so many of us, has heard about the possible virtues of olive oil. Even though it is full of fat, it is the kind of fat that may, in fact, help us improve our cholesterol level.

Indeed, without the help of a class like Everson took, many of us are in the dark when it comes to understanding fully the explosion of information that has rocked the media recently regarding fats in our diet. Some types of fat, in excess, are deadly contributors to heart disease, this country's number one killer. Others, if you listen to their publicity makers, are godsends. Monounsaturated? Polyunsaturated? What does it all mean? Clearly, which fats you choose to eat—or to avoid—make somewhat of a difference when it comes to your weight loss plans or heart disease risk. Read on, and take a look at the different types of fat, as well as a whole new breed known as fake fats.

WHAT ARE FATS?

Before we look into the cornucopia of oils and fats that we can choose to include in our daily diet, let's take a quick look at what fats are.

Fats are organic chemical compounds made up of fatty acids and glycerol (a colorless liquid). The fatty acids are chains of carbon atoms that have varying amounts of hydrogen or oxygen attached. (The amount of hydrogen usually determines how "good" or "bad" a fat may be for you.) In food, as well as in our bodies, fatty acids combine with molecules of glycerol. This combination is known as glyceride. Have you heard of triglycerides? Doctors often test our blood for the level of triglycerides. A triglyceride is three fatty acid molecules attached to one glycerol molecule. There are also monoglycerides (one fatty acid molecule attached to one glycerol molecule) and diglycerides (two fatty acid molecules attached to one glycerol molecule). It is the type of fatty acid involved and the number of hydrogen atoms involved that make a fat saturated, monounsaturated, or polyunsaturated. (We'll go over those momentarily.)

In the small intestine, during digestion, the body converts most eaten fat into triglycerides. Then the triglycerides are transported across the intestinal wall and carried throughout the body. What is needed by the body gets used and is burned off as expended calories. But—dieters beware—what is not needed gets stored in the body's fatty tissue, available if ever needed for energy. For overweight people, however, this just becomes an excess store of fat that is never called upon. When excess carbohydrates or protein are eaten, they are also transformed into triglycerides and stored in the fatty tissue.

With so much of the population overweight—efficiently storing those trigylcerides—is it really necessary for us to include fats in our daily diet? First, since fats are a component of so many foods, it would be difficult to cut them out completely. And, in fact, we do need fat in our diet—but much less than most people consume.

Fat is necessary for energy, and a little fat—much less than most people carry on their frames—is required to insulate and cushion the body. The fat you eat also helps you absorb vitamins A, D, E, and K, which are fat soluble.

You require some fat because your body cannot make linoleic acid, one of the essential fatty acids. But linoleic acid deficiency is very rare; it has been observed only among hospital patients who were fed intravenously with foods containing no fat. The deficiency, which is marked by scaly skin, hair loss, and impaired wound healing, show us another reason fats are important in the diet.

However, the majority of Americans eat a diet that is more than 40 percent fat. All the fat you actually need each day from the food you eat is about the equivalent of one tablespoon of polyunsaturated fat (definition to follow). That translates into three to six grams of linoleic acid. One tablespoon of vegetable oil or margarine easily contains that amount.

When we overload on fat, there are consequences. As I've described throughout this book, excess dietary fat has been irrefutably linked to heart attack, stroke, certain types of cancer, gallstones, indigestion, and perhaps arthritis (because of the strain extra weight puts on joints).

TYPES OF FAT

Most of us probably never thought the advertising industry would become our nutrition instructors. However, their product campaigns regarding monounsaturated, polyunsaturated, and other types of fats—and the virtues or liabilities of each—have been bombarding us from magazine ads and product labels for the last few years. Some of this information is relevant; however, many consumers admit to being nothing less than confused by this small-print jargon.

There really are important differences between fats. A fat is saturated if no hydrogen atoms are missing from the string of molecules that is the fatty acid. Saturated fats come from animal foods like meat, fish, poultry, milk, butter, and cheese. Some vegetable fats—palm, coconut, palm kernel—are also saturated. Saturated fats have been shown to increase blood cholesterol levels.

Monounsaturated fats have one pair of hydrogen atoms missing from the fatty acid chain. Monounsaturated fats come from olive oil, canola (also called rapeseed) oil, peanuts, walnuts, and sesame seeds. Some monounsaturated fats have been shown to raise the good part (the high-density lipoproteins, or HDLs) of blood cholesterol without raising total blood cholesterol.

Polyunsaturated fats have at least two pairs of hydrogen atoms missing from the fatty acid chain. Polyunsaturated fats come from vegetable oils like cottonseed oil, corn oil, sunflower oil, safflower oil, and soybean oil. These fats have been shown to help lower both the good parts (the HDLs) and the bad parts (the low-density lipoproteins, or LDLs) of the blood cholesterol.

There has also been much news in the media lately about hydrogenated and partially hydrogenated fats. Many people, though, admit they are unsure what these are. Actually, hydrogenation starts with a nice unsaturated fat and makes it saturated. Hydrogenation is the process of adding hydrogen molecules to monounsaturated or polyunsaturated fatty acids. The liquid oils used become more saturated with hydrogen and are changed to a semi-solid form. Margarine is made from hydrogenated oils.

Some recent studies have pointed out that the type of fatty acid created by the hydrogenation process may be a cholesterol raiser. A report in the *New England Journal of Medicine* showed that some of these acids, called trans-fatty acids, may raise bad (LDL) cholesterol while lowering good (HDL) cholesterol.

When using hydrogenated foods (hydrogenated oils, etc., are listed on product ingredient lists), simply treat them as if they were saturated fats. (Table 13.1 shows the breakdown of many types of oils and fats.)

Dieters, beware again! Even though saturated, monounsaturated, polyunsaturated, and hydrogenated fats play different roles in our bodies, all fats contain the same (high) amount of calories. Fats contain about 9 calories per gram. That translates to about 100 to 120 calories per tablespoon. Of course, it's a positive step to choose polyunsaturated or monounsaturated fats whenever possible, but don't forget your goal should be to lower your fat intake to well below 30 percent of overall calories.

FATHOMING FAKE FATS

As if most people don't have enough trouble keeping straight all

Table 13.1. The Fat Content of Fats and Oils

Fat or Oil	Milligrams of Cholesterol Per Tablespoon	Percentage of Saturated Fat	Percentage of Monounsaturated Fat	Percentage of Polyunsaturated Fat	Percentage of Other Fats*
Canola Oil	0	7%	56%	33%	4%
Safflower Oil	0	9%	12%	75%	4%
Walnut Oil	0	9%	23%	63%	5%
Sunflower Oil	0	10%	20%	66%	4%
Corn Oil	0	13%	24%	59%	4%
Olive Oil	0	14%	74%	8%	4%
Sesame Oil	0	14%	40%	42%	4%
Soybean Oil	0	14%	23%	58%	5%
Margarine, Soft Tub	0	14%	14%	50%	22%
Margarine, Stick	0	15%	37%	25%	23%
Peanut Oil	0	17%	46%	32%	5%
Cottonseed Oil	0	26%	18%	52%	4%
Chicken Fat	11	30%	45%	21%	4%
Lard (Pork)	12	40%	45%	11%	4%
Palm Oil	0	49%	37%	9%	5%
Beef Tallow	14	50%	42%	4%	4%
Butter	33	62%	29%	4%	5%
Cocoa Butter	0	60%	33%	3%	4%
Palm-Kernel Oil	0	81%	11%	2%	6%
Coconut Oil	0	87%	6%	2%	5%

*The saturated, monounsaturated, and polyunsaturated fatty acids don't add up to 100 percent because other minor fat compounds are present.

Source: U.S. Department of Agriculture Handbook No. 8-4.

the kinds of fats found naturally in foods, now we have a whole new group of fats to contend with: Fake fats. This new genre was first introduced to the marketplace as Simplesse. Its patent is held by the NutraSweet Company. Like NutraSweet, Simplesse is not sold solo but is used as an ingredient in other products. Fake fats can give foods the same texture as fats without the fat and without as many calories. There are now many fake fats on the drawing board and in various stages of development. Here are just five examples:

- DDM (dialkyl dihexadecylmatlonate), under development by Frito-Lay, is a synthetic fat and may be appropriate for fried foods and snacks.

- EPG (esterified propoxylated glycerol), being developed by ARCO Chemical Company, is non-caloric and can substitute for fat or oil.

- Modified Protein Texturizers, Kraft's addition to the fake-fat market, is similar to Simplesse. The process for both begins with proteins that have been changed in physical form.

- Olestra is a calorie-free fat substitute being developed by Procter & Gamble. It is a combination of sugar and vegetable oil in a new molecule containing the taste and texture of fat. The FDA is reviewing it.

- Tatca (trialkoxytricarballylate), bread and pastry manufacturer CPC International's entry into the fat-substitute race, has no calories and is an oil-like compound.

Do I really need to tell you that man-made ingredients with names like "trialkoxytricarballylate" or terms such as "oil-like" have no place in the diet of people who are trying to follow a natural foods diet? Anyone recommending a natural foods diet, which has been proven healthful, would say to avoid these new artificial ingredients. There have been no tests to show what these compounds do inside your body over the long term.

Even people who don't recommend ditching all artificial additives express concern about fake fats. Lisa Lefferts, a staff scientist for the Center for Science in the Public Interest, has asked the FDA to monitor closely a group of people who follow a diet using fake fats. Normally the FDA tests only small amounts of such ingredients, she said, but "we're asking for a somewhat broader view because [fake fats] would be consumed in larger amounts than any other additive currently used."

The only fairly long-term studies done on, for example, Olestra, were on rats. These showed some evidence of pituitary tumors and possibly pre-cancerous liver changes, said Lefferts. Another concern regarding fake fats is their impact on fat-soluble vitamins.

"If fake fats are not absorbed," said American Dietetic Association spokesperson Margaret Wing-Peterson, "what will it do to those vitamins? Will it tie them and reduce their absorption?" The *American Journal of Clinical Nutrition* has reported that vitamins such as A and E are not absorbed well in Olestra and some other fake fats.

The California Dietetic Association recently sent out an alert that fake fats may not even offer that much benefit when it comes to calorie reduction in the diet.

Simplesse, they wrote, "is not the miracle ingredient one might imagine where calories are concerned. Dieters should beware: The caloric savings are not as substantial as weight watchers may first be led to believe. A four-ounce serving of an ice cream-like product made with the fat substitute contains 120 calories. Regular ice cream is about 150 calories per serving."

Simplesse is so named, the NutraSweet Company reported, because it makes things so "simple." However, it really is simple for people wanting to eat a natural foods diet to find replacements for the same kind of foods without filling themselves with refined sugar, additives, calories, or fat. In the case of a frozen dessert, for example, why not choose a non-fat frozen yogurt that is sweetened with honey or unrefined fructose? In that case, you are actually adding to your health. You are eating something low in calories, with no fat, and high in calcium. There are many brands available that can help you make those types of switches.

Fake fats are just one of a multitude of "fake" ingredients that are being unleashed on us. As the Mayo Clinic warned in their journal, however, be wary of such additives:

"This is an era of high-tech food, but that doesn't mean you should eat indiscriminately and rely on artificial processing to keep you healthy. A proper diet involves more than leaving 'bad things' out. It means taking 'good things' in.

"The proliferation of substitutes may soon mean you can eat a completely synthetic meal from appetizer to dessert. Yet the long-range health effects of these products are unknown. Questions also remain about how artificial foods mix with medications and other substances in the body."

Although the possible dangers of "high-tech food" are of great concern, we shouldn't let them distract us from the fundamental issue of fats and oils in our diet. While some fat is indeed necessary for good health, the fact is that most Americans consume perhaps twice as much as they really need. Our goal should be to reduce that total fat consumption, and especially consumption of saturated and hydrogenated fats and oils, by eating a natural, nutritionally balanced diet. That way, we can avoid turning our bodies into chemistry experiments, and at the same time make an investment in a healthier future.

14

Cholesterol

Years ago, when Mom (or Dad, or the best cook in the family) got out the cookbook to whip up a meatloaf, a chicken pot pie, or a bowl of homemade mashed potatoes for dinner, there probably wasn't a scientific breakdown of protein, carbohydrates, cholesterol, sodium, total fat, saturated fat, polyunsaturated fat, and monounsaturated fat at the bottom of each recipe.

However, that's just what the American Heart Association has tagged on to those and hundreds of other recipes in the fifth edition of the *American Heart Association Cookbook*. With all the numerical breakdowns, those recipes—as well as recipes in lots of other cookbooks—sometimes read as much like stock market reports as instructions for making tuna casserole or tomato soup. However, with all the studies that have linked diet to the promotion and prevention of serious diseases, today even a moderately health-conscious family clearly has a valid need for a lot more information than how many teaspoons of onion powder or how many cups of flour go into a recipe.

But what does all that information really mean? Many people who are trying to monitor their consumption of cholesterol readily admit that they are not sure exactly what cholesterol is. Others complain that they can't keep straight the difference between HDLs and LDLs, and they chide themselves for not knowing what those letters stand for. (They stand for high-density lipoproteins and low-density lipoproteins.)

WHAT IS CHOLESTEROL?

"This new fifth edition of the *American Heart Association Cookbook* comes eighteen years after the first edition. Times have changed. In those days we suspected that high blood cholesterol was a major cause of heart attack; today, we know it," writes Dr. Rodman D. Starke, senior vice president of scientific affairs for the American Heart Association, as the very first lines of the 643-page book.

Most people almost would have had to have been visiting another planet during the last decade not to have heard the news that cutting cholesterol in the diet will likely cut the risk for heart disease and heart attack. But many people say it would be much easier for them to stick to a cholesterol-cutting regimen if they understood just what cholesterol is and what it does inside their bodies.

Cholesterol is a wax-like, white substance that is a component of every cell in the body. The cholesterol that your body manufactures does a lot of good.

Cholesterol plays a role in cell wall development throughout the body. In addition, the body's sex hormones could not be produced without cholesterol. These hormones include estrogen, progesterone, and testosterone. Bile acids are also made from cholesterol. Bile is a yellow, bitter fluid secreted by the liver and found in the gall bladder. It helps in the digestion of fats. Adrenal hormones are made from cholesterol. These hormones produce the "fight or flight" anxiety response in human beings. Vitamin D, needed for the metabolism of calcium, is synthesized from cholesterol.

So, if cholesterol has so many important functions in the body, why has virtually everyone tried to reduce or eliminate their consumption of it? Actually, the body is so good at producing cholesterol on its own that it makes all that it needs. People don't need the extra cholesterol they get from their diets. And the rub, of course, is that if we have elevated amounts of cholesterol in our blood, we become much more likely to develop heart disease or have heart attacks.

Cholesterol is found only in foods of animal origin. There is no cholesterol in vegetable products. However, saturated fat contributes greatly to the creation of cholesterol in our bodies. Even a food with no cholesterol may contain saturated fat. Ingredients high in saturated fat include palm oil, coconut oil, and cocoa butter. When an animal product, like meat, is eaten, some people think they can trim away the cholesterol. Unfortunately, that's not so. You can trim away some of the visible white fat, but cholesterol is also in the muscles of animals, so it's in the marbling of meat and cannot be cut away.

Studies regarding the effect of cholesterol on the body have become more frequent in recent years, but they are not new. Scientists have been studying cholesterol and its relationship to coronary heart disease for almost 100 years. At about the turn of the century, researchers observed that animals fed high-cholesterol diets developed lesions that looked like the atherosclerosis found in humans.

Atherosclerosis is a form of arteriosclerosis, which is a progressive disease of the arteries. Arteriosclerosis occurs when fatty substances, which are mainly cholesterol, gradually stick to the inner lining of the body's arteries. Eventually, blockage can occur. When an artery supplying the heart is blocked, a heart attack can occur. If an artery supplying the brain is blocked, then a stroke can occur.

Although the first studies involving cholesterol were done early in the twentieth century, the frequency of tests did not start increasing until a few decades ago. One of the most informative studies ever conducted on the subject is the Framingham (Massachusetts) Heart Study. This ongoing study has examined heart disease, first in men and later in whole families, since 1948. The study has shown that men who have cholesterol levels of 260 milligrams per deciliter of blood and above have had three times the number of heart attacks as men whose blood cholesterol levels averaged 195. Studies have shown that, although coronary heart disease has other risk factors, such as smoking and hypertension, cholesterol is clearly the primary culprit.

High blood cholesterol levels have been linked to heart disease, but does that mean that lowering the amount of cholesterol you eat will reduce your risk of developing the disease? The Lipid Research Clinics Coronary Primary Prevention Trial, conducted in 1984, was a landmark study because it was one of the first to show a clear link between eating less cholesterol and preventing heart attacks. The study of almost 4,000 men concluded that a 10-percent reduction of blood cholesterol through diet led to an almost 20-percent reduction in fatal and non-fatal heart attacks.

Lots of other studies have proven such a link. The American Heart Association might almost as well be called the American Cholesterol Reduction Association at this point. Their literature, which used to stress a number of precursors to heart disease, now mainly trumpets cholesterol as a culprit.

"Scientific evidence implicating high blood cholesterol as a major risk factor for heart and blood vessel disease is overwhelming," they wrote in a recent advisory. "It comes from countless epidemiologic studies [studies of large populations all over the world] and from clinical, genetic, and animal studies. These studies not only confirm the link between high blood cholesterol and the development of atherosclerosis but also strongly suggest that reducing the blood cholesterol level will reduce the risk of heart attack. This is true not only for middle-aged men with high blood cholesterol, but also for younger and older men, for women, and for people with just mildly elevated blood cholesterol."

While some studies have shown that what we eat affects blood cholesterol levels, some recent ones have shown that even what we *don't* eat can make a difference. A study, for example, reported in a 1991 edition of the *Journal of School Health* showed that children who consistently skip breakfast have significantly higher blood cholesterol levels than those who don't.

The eating habits of over 500 students between age nine and nineteen were analyzed. Those who regularly skipped breakfast had an average blood cholesterol level of 172, above the 165 national average for children in that age range. The children who regularly ate breakfast, however, had average blood cholesterol levels of 149. The fiber that the children ate at breakfast, researchers said, was probably responsible for the difference in cholesterol levels. Fiber has been shown to help lower blood cholesterol levels.

JUST WHAT ARE HDLS AND LDLS?

Many people are slowly realizing that cholesterol is manufactured by our bodies as well as being present in many of the foods we eat. However, lots of those same people are quick to admit they lose the scent after that point and get terribly lost on the cholesterol trail.

"I think I understand a little bit about cholesterol and which foods have it," said Mark Herman, a San Diego carpenter. "But when it comes to those letters—LDLs and HDLs—I just have no idea what they mean. I know one is supposed to be good and the other bad, but I'm not sure which is which."

High-density lipoproteins (HDLs) and low-density lipoproteins (LDLs) are two of four types of lipoproteins that carry cholesterol back and forth between the liver and the cells in the blood stream. Lipoproteins are minute globular shapes that have an outer coating of fat and protein. Cholesterol and triglycerides (a chemical form of fat) travel within the tiny globes.

Triglyceride levels within the body are often measured along with cholesterol. However, elevated triglyceride levels alone are usually not thought to be a coronary heart disease risk factor. When they are elevated, though, it is usually a sign that a patient has a high blood cholesterol level, obesity, or some other problem that can lead to heart disease.

HDLs remove cholesterol from the cells and cleanly transport it to the liver for processing. HDLs have thus been dubbed "good" cholesterol. LDLs sometimes leave deposits of cholesterol in the arteries when they are making their journey to the liver. This can lead to plaque buildup. Therefore, when people try to lower the level of their blood cholesterol, they should be attempting to lower only the LDL level. Coronary risk can be lowered either by lowering LDL levels or by increasing HDL levels. An easy trick to remember the difference is to think that you always want to "take the high (density) road." That's the good one. You certainly wouldn't want to take the low road when it comes to cholesterol. (For more details on how you can eat to lower your LDL levels, see Chapters 2, 13, and 15.)

CHOLESTEROL BY THE NUMBERS

About 32 percent of adults reported that they knew their cholesterol levels in 1990, about twice as many as the year before, according to Gallup surveys. Physicians recommend that all adults know their cholesterol levels and those of their children over age five, many of whom show early—and preventable—heart disease symptoms.

Studies have shown that the people at the greatest risk for developing heart disease are those who have a blood cholesterol level of at least 240 milligrams per deciliter (mg/dl) of blood. Some risk is believed to exist at levels of 200 to 239 mg/dl. Those considered to be at low risk have levels below 200 mg/dl. However, those numbers are not written in stone. Many researchers suggest that although the numbers below 200 are acceptable, the truly optimal level for cholesterol is a person's age plus 100. Because of the important difference between lipoproteins, make sure any blood cholesterol test you take includes a determination of your HDL level. Normal HDL levels for adults are 45 to 50 mg/dl for men and 50 to 60 mg/dl for women. Higher levels, in the area of 70 to 80 mg/dl, are desirable. Even if your total blood cholesterol level is relatively low, if your HDL level is *under* 35 mg/dl, you would be considered at greater risk for heart disease.

We now know it's wise to be concerned about cholesterol. So keep in touch with your cholesterol count. And don't get swept away by all the advertising hype about cholesterol. Just because a package proclaims "No cholesterol" doesn't mean that what's inside it is good for you. Read the fine print, and use sources like this book to learn the facts about what you can do to get—and keep—your cholesterol level down where you want it.

15

Fiber

Health Valley is the country's largest health food manufacturer. They have hundreds of products available in health food stores and supermarkets. You'd think it would be just that variety that helped ensure their success. Not so, according to Harry Urist, one of the company's directors. Although Health Valley has been in business for more than twenty years, the real explosion in supermarket sales occurred in the late 1980s, when the national oat bran craze hit. Because of that one ingredient, Urist said, supermarkets started really increasing Health Valley orders—orders that have just kept growing. Urist's, of course, wasn't the only company to profit from the oat bran boom. According to Nielsen Marketing Research, 1987's first-quarter supermarket sales of products containing oat bran were $7.2 million, but by 1989—after all the publicity about oat bran's possible health benefits—first-quarter sales had soared to $71.5 million.

The millions of mothers who decades ago served their children big bowls of oatmeal, which is one-third oat bran, probably never dreamed that in that gooey glob was a dynamic wonder food of the future. The publicity about oat bran has helped make fiber a household word. By being possibly linked to the lowering of cholesterol and the prevention of cancer, it started a fiber fad in this country that has led to frantic shopper searches for products with rice bran, wheat bran, soy fiber, and many other types of bran and fiber. But, besides increasing food manufacturers' profit margins, just what can bran and fiber really do for us? Can they really help prevent disease? Many shoppers who choose products with labels that boast "high fiber" admit they are not really sure what the big deal is about. Let's take a look.

WHAT IS FIBER?

First let's examine just what dietary fiber is and then take a look at some of the reasons so many people have become devoted "fiber followers." In the past, fiber was often referred to as roughage. Although many people are running to eat as much fiber as possible, fiber is actually the part of plant materials that our bodies cannot digest. Their fibrous texture causes these foods to act like a kitchen broom, sweeping wastes out of the colon and intestines. Fiber is classified as a carbohydrate, but since it is not digested, it contributes almost no calories.

The words "fiber" and "bran" sometimes are used interchangeably. However, bran is a type of fiber. Bran is the outer layers of a cereal grain like oat, wheat, or rye. Much of the hoopla surrounding bran is due to the fact that most of the nutrients in the cereal grain are in its high-fiber bran.

Fiber is often divided into two categories: Soluble and insoluble. Insoluble fiber—the thread or wood-like part of the husks and shells of fiber-rich foods—promotes regularity and is the type of fiber that may be connected to preventing colon and rectal cancer. Good sources of insoluble fiber are whole grains, nuts, vegetables, dried beans, and peas.

Soluble fiber—found in the cell walls of fiber-rich foods—is the newcomer on the fiber research block. Only recently have studies shown that the digestive and absorptive effects of soluble fiber may help lower blood cholesterol levels. This is because soluble fiber may bind bile acids in the intestine, preventing their re-absorption, and preventing cholesterol and fat absorption. Increasing the consumption of foods containing soluble fiber has also been shown to help diabetics control their blood glucose levels. Soluble fiber is found in whole-grain oats, oat bran, some fruits, dried beans, and legumes.

WHAT ARE THE BENEFITS OF CONSUMING FIBER?

First of all, before we even examine any of the information about fiber's possible link to cancer prevention or cholesterol reduction, there is good news for dieters. Foods containing fiber are very filling, and yet—a true dieter's dream—fiber itself, since it is not digested, adds virtually no calories to your diet. So, if you fill up on whole-grain cereals, crackers, fruits, and vegetables, you are, indeed, filling up without adding many calories or much fat to your diet.

As far as all the research into oat bran and other fibrous foods goes, it started innocently in the 1970s. Dr. Dennis Burkitt, an English physician who took care of rural Africans for twenty years, reported that he had rarely seen cases of heart disease, colon cancer, gallstones, ulcers, or hemorrhoids among his patients. Burkitt reported that he thought this was related to the ample amounts of fiber they ate each day.

This inspired scientists in the United States to begin research. The news in the mid-1980s, of course, was that eating oat bran could lower blood cholesterol. Oat bran was lucky. It got all the publicity. Later studies showed that rice bran, wheat bran, and other brans also were effective. The resulting hoopla in supermarkets was because some of the first studies showed that cholesterol was reduced by as much as 15 to 20 percent by adding moderate amounts of oat bran to the diet.

Later studies, particularly one from Harvard University that was reported in the *New England Journal of Medicine*, showed that in order to lower cholesterol a low-fat diet must also be eaten. In 1990, for instance, Syracuse University researchers studied seventy-one men and women with high cholesterol and found that a low-fat diet combined with 1.7 ounces a day of oat bran or 1.5 ounces a day of cold oat bran cereal reduced cholesterol by 10 to 17 percent.

Researcher Becky Reeves of Baylor College of Medicine in Texas has found that people with the highest cholesterol levels have much to gain from eating oat bran and other fibrous foods. Those with cholesterol levels over 240 show the most dramatic drops when switching to a diet that includes about 3.5 ounces of fibrous bran a day. That translates to one serving of oat bran and five oat bran muffins a day. "If you can eat that much each day," Reeves told the Associated Press, "you may reduce your cholesterol by almost 20 percent. And it's a lot cheaper than using cholesterol-reducing drugs."

A study at Louisiana State University showed that rice bran helped lower the cholesterol of people who were borderline high (190 to 230). That study confirmed the results of one done by the University of California at Davis and earlier research performed in Australia. By supplementing their diets with rice bran in a ten-week controlled diet program, LSU study participants lowered their cholesterol by 7 percent.

Wheat bran has been shown to protect the colon in a number of ways, according to much research, including recent studies by Dr. Bandaru S. Reddy of the American Health Foundation in New York. Since wheat bran increases the weight of the stool, it can dilute the concentration of secondary acids. These acids cannot then help cancers develop, because the bran binds them. Studies done more recently at the University of Arizona support Reddy's research.

WHAT ABOUT FIBER?

The important research regarding fiber has made health agencies jump to attention in announcing healthful amounts to consume. The American Dietetic Association, the American Heart Association, and the National Cancer Institute recommend consuming about thirty to thirty-five grams of dietary fiber per day. However, according to research from Tufts University, the average American consumes only eleven to seventeen grams per day. Because too much fiber can cause gas or digestive problems, no one recommends consuming more than fifty grams per day, and the National Cancer Institute recommends eating no more than forty grams.

Since much of fiber acts as a sponge, dietitians recommend increasing your water intake when you increase your fiber intake. And it's important, if your system is not used to large amounts of fiber, which is not digestible, to increase your fiber intake slowly.

The Mayo Clinic advises increasing fiber in the diet over a six-week period.

Increasing fiber is not difficult. It can be a delicious mission. Do read labels. Many labels, especially on foods that tout their bran or oat ingredients, will list how much fiber is in each serving. An especially good fiber source would contain three or more grams of dietary fiber per serving. And do read labels carefully. They can be out to sell you, rather than inform you.

As I was writing this chapter, for example, I trotted into my kitchen to look at the labels on the three oat, fiber, or rice bran cereals in the cupboard. The one I had for breakfast that day said it had five grams of dietary fiber per serving. Another claimed to have fifteen grams. (There can be that big a difference between products.) I left the kitchen thinking the fifteen-gram-per-serving cereal was obviously a better fiber choice. However, I had to rub my eyes, return to the kitchen, and squint at the labels again. The fifteen grams was actually the amount of oat bran per serving. In smaller print below, it listed that the product contained three grams per serving of actual dietary fiber—the result of eating all that oat bran.

When it comes to your choice of bread, also watch out for label double-talk. A label may announce the product contains bran, but you should be looking for breads that have whole-wheat or whole-grain flour as the first-listed (meaning main) ingredient. Many breads that brag about bran are made with enriched or unbleached flours, which are not good sources of fiber.

What can you do to add fiber to your diet?

In addition to eating high-fiber cereals, you can sprinkle oat bran into soups and salads. Oat, wheat, or rice bran can also be substituted for up to one-quarter of the flour in a cake, cookie, or bread recipe.

Some foods definitely contain more fiber than others. A carrot contains about twice as much fiber as a stalk of celery. An apple eaten with the skin has about five times the fiber of a piece of watermelon. Pinto beans have about double the fiber of chickpeas. And drop those saltines! Whole-grain crackers have about five times as much fiber as saltines.

Don't think you can eat thirty to thirty-five grams of fiber a day? Following is an example of a day's worth of fibrous foods that could be added to your menu:

Breakfast: 1 medium banana (3 grams fiber); 1 cup high-fiber cereal (3 grams or more).

Lunch: ½ cup baked beans (7 grams); 1 medium pear (4 grams).

Snack: 1 small apple (3 grams); 1 medium bran muffin (3 grams).

Dinner: 1 medium potato with skin (4 grams); ½ cup broccoli (3 grams); 1 slice whole-grain bread (2 grams).

Your total fiber intake for the day would be 32 grams.

Food calculations—even by noted scientists—can be an art rather than a science. The menu suggested above is based on numbers from the Mayo Clinic. Table 15.1, which comes from the *Journal of the American Dietetic Association* and looks at fiber values for many foods, gives counts that sometimes vary slightly from the Mayo Clinic numbers. But you will certainly get the general idea of which foods are high in fiber and which are low.

Table 15.1. Foods and the Amount of Dietary Fiber They Contain

Food	Amount	Grams of Dietary Fiber	Calories
Fruits			
Apple (with skin)	1 medium	3.5	81
Banana	1 medium	2.4	105
Cantaloupe	¼ melon	1.0	30
Cherries, sweet	10	1.2	49
Peach (with skin)	1	1.9	37
Pear (with skin)	½ large	3.1	61
Prunes	3	3.0	60
Raisins	¼ cup	3.1	108
Raspberries	½ cup	3.1	35
Strawberries	1 cup	3.0	45
Orange	1 medium	2.6	62
Vegetables, Cooked			
Asparagus, cut	½ cup	1.0	15

Adapted from a critcal review of food fiber analysis and data by E. Lanza and R.R. Butron. *Journal of the American Dietetic Association* 86:732. 1986.

Food	Amount	Grams of Dietary Fiber	Calories
Beans, string, green	½ cup	1.6	16
Broccoli	½ cup	2.2	20
Brussels sprouts	½ cup	2.3	28
Parsnips	½ cup	2.7	51
Potato (with skin)	1 medium	2.5	106
Spinach	½ cup	2.1	21
Sweet potato	½ medium	1.7	80
Turnip	½ cup	1.6	17
Zucchini	½ cup	1.8	11

Vegetables, Raw

Celery, diced	½ cup	1.1	10
Cucumber	½ cup	0.4	8
Lettuce, sliced	1 cup	0.9	7
Mushrooms, sliced	½ cup	0.9	10
Tomato	1 medium	1.5	20
Spinach	1 cup	1.2	8

Legumes

Baked beans	½ cup	8.8	155
Dried peas, cooked	½ cup	4.7	115
Kidney beans, cooked	½ cup	7.3	110
Lima beans, cooked	½ cup	4.5	64
Lentils, cooked	½ cup	3.7	97
Navy beans, cooked	½ cup	6.0	112

Breads, Pastas, and Flours

Bagels	1 bagel	0.6	145
Bran muffins	1 muffin	2.5	104
French bread	1 slice	0.7	102
Oatmeal bread	1 slice	0.5	63

Food	Amount	Grams of Dietary Fiber	Calories
Pumpernickel bread	1 slice	1.0	66
Whole wheat bread	1 slice	1.4	61
Rice, brown, cooked	½ cup	1.0	97
Spaghetti, cooked	½ cup	1.1	155
Nuts and Seeds			
Almonds	10 nuts	1.1	79
Peanuts	10 nuts	1.4	105
Filberts	10 nuts	0.8	54
Popcorn, popped	1 cup	1.0	54
Breakfast Cereals			
All-Bran	⅓ cup	8.5	71
Bran Buds	⅓ cup	7.9	73
Bran Chex	⅔ cup	4.6	91
Corn Bran	⅔ cup	5.4	98
40% Bran-type	¾ cup	4.0	93
Raisin Bran-type	¾ cup	4.0	115
Shredded wheat	⅔ cup	2.6	102
Oatmeal, regular, quick and instant, cooked	¾ cup	1.6	108
Cornflakes	1¼ cup	0.3	110

Fiber is clearly a dietary friend. It can help lower cholesterol. It can aid in a weight-loss program. It can help prevent certain types of cancer. And, it can provide all of these benefits through delicious foods that can be easily incorporated in your daily menus. What more reason do you need to add fiber to your diet?

16

Additives and Artificial Ingredients

Over 3,000 additives are added to the foods we eat. An average supermarket holds 18,000 items, of which over 15,000 are processed. I have to admit I thought I knew my way around the food jungles we call supermarkets. I have always been a food label reader. However, it wasn't until I started intense research for my 1991 book, *Turn Your Supermarket Into a Health Food Store: The Brand Name Guide to Shopping for a Better Diet*, that I got a surprising education about the additives, chemicals, and artificial ingredients in our foods. Since then my education has continued, and I would like to share with you some of the most interesting points that I don't think any truly health-concerned shopper would want to be without.

Some people might ask: Shouldn't we trust food manufacturers or the Food and Drug Administration, which oversees what additives are used in foods, about the foods we buy in our supermarkets or health food stores? To a certain extent, we should be confident. However, there are some key points to be aware of that form the basis of why more and more people choose to avoid foods prepared with additives or preservatives.

Additives are usually in foods in such small amounts that perhaps you think you really don't eat much of them. However, Michael Jacobson, Ph.D., executive director of the Center for

Science in the Public Interest, cites studies showing that the average American consumes about five pounds of additives a year. When you think about the small amount of additives used in most foods, you can see just how many additives you would have to be eating—and how often—to add up to five pounds. When you include sugar (the food-processing industry's most used additive), that number jumps to 135 pounds per year.

The FDA declares some additives Generally Recognized as Safe (GRAS). Many other additives are declared GRAS but with a notation that further study is needed. Additives are never given permanent approval. The FDA and the Food Safety and Inspection Service (FSIS) of the United States Department of Agriculture (USDA) are supposed to review the safety of approved additives continually to determine if approvals should be modified or withdrawn.

Of course, you don't receive information that an additive is Generally Recognized as Safe but still judged to need further testing when you see such an additive listed on a product label. Why fill yourself and your family with a substance that still needs more testing and is fairly easy to avoid? And, most important, why consume an additive that today may be declared GRAS but that in two or ten or twenty years is thrown off the GRAS list and out of the food supply because its true status as a carcinogen finally becomes known? You may end up with years of an additive under your belt, in your blood stream or clogged in some artery, before the true dangers are discovered or acknowledged by the FDA.

And, of course, this has happened. That was the case with the popular artificial sweeteners cyclamate and xylitol and with many other additives. There is a more recent example of an additive we have been ingesting for decades that the FDA eventually banned. In January 1990, the FDA announced the delisting of FD&C Red Lake No. 3 (an artificial coloring) from foods, drugs, and cosmetics.

Studies showed that high dosages of FD&C No. 3 have triggered thyroid changes that could cause cancer. "FD&C Red No. 3 is a proven carcinogen. The FDA has taken twenty-nine years to make a final decision," complained attorney William Schultz of Public Citizen to the media when the ban was imposed. (Public Citizen was founded by Ralph Nader.)

And yet, while some uses of FD&C Red No. 3 have been banned, we still may be ingesting the questionable additive while final steps are taken by the FDA.

Food Processing: The Magazine of the Food Industry recently advised its readers: "The recent ban involves only the provisional approval of the food color in lake (powdered) form and does not yet disapprove 'permanently' listed uses of the food dye form in ingested drugs and foods (e.g., maraschino cherries). However, the lengthy legal process to delist all applications will be initiated by FDA."

It's not as if there are no natural alternatives to additives like FD&C Red Lake No. 3, or virtually any other chemically derived additive. Japanese researchers, for example, recently introduced in the United States a coloring derived from red cabbage. Since it is made from natural vegetable juice, it doesn't even need FDA approval. It is already being used in salad dressing, juice, and hard candy. It also may soon be used in tomato and barbecue sauces, pudding, and yogurt. Food magazines are predicting the red cabbage extract will be a major food ingredient in the next decade.

WHAT DOES ADDITIVE "X" PLUS ADDITIVE "Y" EQUAL?

Besides eating maraschino cherries, gelatin, dyed pistachio nuts (all of which contain Red Lake No. 3), or other foods that may contain additives the FDA is trying to get rid of, many experts point out, there may be serious implications to ingesting the rainbow of additives and preservatives available that the FDA has not even considered.

Although the FDA may look into the effect a single additive has on a test animal, many of us consume many different additives every day or even within a given meal. How do these additives act together? This is a scary scenario that, as we munch away on thousands of additives a year, no one has yet fully studied. And because of the sheer number of additives and possible combinations, adequate studies are probably not even possible.

Dr. Arnold Fox, a well-known Beverly Hills cardiologist and former professor of medicine at the University of California at Irvine, articulated this widely-held concern in *Immune for Life*, a book he wrote with his son Barry: "We don't know what happens when the chemicals get together inside your body. Chemical A in your ice cream may be relatively harmless by itself. So might Chemical B in your fast-food french fries. But what happens when the two chemicals meet in your blood stream or liver? Do they ignore each other? Do they combine? Does A convert B into a more dangerous form?"

MUST PACKAGED FOODS CONTAIN ADDITIVES?

Many food manufacturers argue that to flavor or preserve their foods they must include additives. In fact, they will often slip you messages to this effect—to comfort you, no doubt—within the ingredients list. After an ominous chemical name, for instance, they might include "to preserve freshness" or "as a softener" or "as a flavor enhancer."

Don't be taken in by such attempts. Manufacturers of packaged health food have been proving for years that all of those chemicals and preservatives, are, in fact, most often not needed. And many of their products, once found only in health food stores, are now moving in full force into our supermarkets. They are not hiding in the "diet" aisles, either. Extensive interviews I conducted with supermarket chains nationwide show that most chains simply "mainstream" such all-around healthful products throughout the store.

And many major brands turn out completely natural, healthful products, too. During my many hours of aisle-to-aisle combat research on the floors of supermarkets, I cannot tell you how many times I found within a group of nationally known competitors just one product that contained no sugar, no preservatives, and no chemicals, although almost all the other brands in the category did contain them. This proves that the chemicals and preservatives are not a necessity.

Would you, for instance, have to think twice about buying Orville Redenbacher's Gourmet Natural Flavor Microwave Popping Corn or Newman's Own All Natural Flavor Microwave Popping Corn? Almost all the other brands of microwave popcorn available have added "to protect flavor" questionable preservatives like BHA, BHT, and TBHQ, which is a particularly troublesome ingredient that contains petroleum-derived butane and took much pushing by manufacturers before FDA approval. As little as a five-gram ingestion has caused death; one gram has resulted in collapse, nausea, vomiting, delirium, and a sense of suffocation. The Redenbacher and Newman's Own brands do not have these preservatives. Are you going to be any less happy with those brands? Will the flavor be noticeably different? Most consumers who buy those products wouldn't think so.

Apparently, Jolly Time, one of the country's top three popcorns, all of a sudden doesn't think so, either. When I wrote my supermarket research book, their popular microwave popcorn contained BHA and BHT. However, during the fall of 1991, Jolly Time sent out press packets to daily newspaper food editors like me, bragging about their change of sentiment concerning making their products more healthful.

In a press release titled "Jolly Time Is Now 100 Percent Natural," American Pop Corn Company announced: "Jolly Time Butter Flavored and Natural Flavor Microwave Pop Corn products will soon be 100 percent all natural with no artificial flavors, colors, or preservatives." It then stated that Jolly Time will no longer contain BHA or BHT.

Interestingly, although another press release in the packet touted Jolly Time as the country's oldest popcorn brand, the company states that it took them until 1991 to conduct tests that showed that preservatives did nothing to improve the product. "Jolly Time was able to make the move to 100 percent all natural after a series of tests showed that these changes did not alter the products' freshness and quality," their release states. Perhaps a truer reason for the switch is the "ring, ring" of cash registers in supermarkets, for the release later states: "Jolly Time is confident that consumers will welcome the change. It matches today's trends and consumers' appetite for natural flavors and fewer product additives and preservatives."

You see? Our opinions, as Jolly Time stated, really make a difference. If we show manufacturers with our food dollars that we want natural foods with no additives, that may be just what we get.

17

Food Labeling

Most of our supermarkets are such confusing promotional jungles that it may be difficult to find the products that are truly healthful. And much of this confusion is the result of unclear, inadequate, or misleading food labels.

First, you should know that until the long-awaited food-labeling reforms of 1992—reforms that won't be effective until May of 1994—not all processed products were required to carry nutritional information on their labels. At this time, some manufacturers do so voluntarily, but they are not required to unless they make a nutritional claim or the product as been enriched (replacing nutrients lost during processing) or fortified (adding nutrients not present in the food's natural state). Only about 55 percent of packaged products carry nutritional labeling. But that number will increase because of new labeling laws, which we will discuss in a moment.

At this time, even when labels do give nutritional information, the consumer must beware of confusing claims. And, when the new laws go into effect, it will still take a wise shopper to select the most nutritional foods available.

CURRENT FOOD LABELING

One source of confusion about current labels is that the same word may have different meanings on different labels:

- Foods labeled "light" (often "lite") are near the top of all product introductions. But light can mean a variety of things. It can mean a product is lower in calories than its original version. It can simply mean it is lighter in taste, texture, color, fat, cholesterol, or sodium. Fortunately, new labeling laws will result in standard definitions for terms like light.

- A product labeled "no salt" or "salt-free" may have other sources of sodium. The American Dietetic Association warns that there are more than seventy different sodium compounds used in food processing. Such ingredients include monosodium glutamate and sodium phosphate. The word "sodium" in any ingredient is a tip-off. That is why it is so important to look at the nutrition-per-serving listings on a food label. The sodium milligrams listed there will tell the true story.

  Nutritionists recommend a limit of 3,000 milligrams of sodium per day. To put this into perspective, we must first be aware that just one teaspoon of salt has 2,300 milligrams. But since most of us never sit down to read our morning paper and enjoy a teaspoonful of salt, what does this mean in terms of the foods we actually eat? Well, if your lunch includes two slices of Eckrich salami, you'd be ingesting 1,200 milligrams of sodium. If dinner includes a serving of Campbell's Home Cookin' Country Vegetable Soup, that would add another 1,070 milligrams. The Weight Watchers Lasagna entrée you might have with your soup would add another 990 milligrams to your sodium count. At a total of 3,260 milligrams of sodium, that puts you over the recommended level after eating only three foods!

  Some current sodium label terms do carry a particular meaning. "Sodium-free" means the product has less than 5 milligrams of sodium per serving. "Low sodium" means 140 milligrams of sodium or less in a serving. "Very low sodium" means 35 milligrams of sodium or less in a serving. "Reduced sodium" means the usual level of sodium in a product has been reduced by at least 75 percent.

- A product labeled "no refined sugar" might have no refined sugar, but it may instead contain other processed sugars such as high-fructose corn syrup.

- A product labeled "high-fiber" is using a term for which, in current labeling, there is no standard definition. As syndicated nutrition writer Lorna Sass has noted, "Your definition of high may be someone else's definition of low." Nutritionists and other experts recommend no less than 20 and up to 35 grams of fiber per day. Foods considered good sources of fiber usually contain 3 or more grams of dietary fiber per serving. Many products claim they are good sources of fiber even though there is barely any bran or fiber in a serving. The FDA recently sent letters to six companies warning them to remove what they called "unsubstantiated" fiber claims.

- "Low cholesterol" and "low fat" can be very misleading terms on current food labels since there are no standard definitions. Low fat is defined only in the dairy aisle, where it means milk with less than 2 percent fat.

We've seen a lot of complex mathematical ways to determine the percentage of fat a food contains. A quicker but different calculation is to think that for every hundred calories of a product you eat, ideally there should be no more than 3 grams of fat. Therefore, if a label reads that a serving of food has 200 calories, there should be no more than 6 grams of fat listed for that serving.

Nutritionists urge you to get no more than 30 percent of your daily calories from fat. As for cholesterol, the American Heart Association and other health organizations suggest no more than 300 milligrams per day.

Knowing how much fat or cholesterol we should eat is one thing, but that may not help when we come across the sea of hype on many products. "Ingredient claims can be more confusing than helpful. Perhaps the best example is the plethora of products marked 'cholesterol-free,' " noted Jean Mayer, president of Tufts University, and Jeanne Goldberg in their syndicated nutrition column. "But are you better off buying a food labeled this way? Not necessarily. The catch is that the product beside it on the shelf that lacks a cholesterol-free tag . . . also may contain no cholesterol."

Some manufacturers promote cholesterol-free versions of foods that barely had any cholesterol to begin with, such as mayonnaise. The regular versions of the country's most popular mayonnaises only contain 5 milligrams of cholesterol per serving. The packages of other products, like peanut butter, proclaim that they are cholesterol-free even though they never had any cholesterol in the first place.

When it comes to fat claims on products, consumers can also be easily duped. Many products are now claiming things like "85 percent fat-free" or "95 percent fat-free." That sounds pretty good, doesn't it? Well, many people don't realize that these descriptions refer to the weight of a fat in a food, not fat calories. The potentially misleading fact is that fat, although high in calories, actually weighs very little.

"Fat labeling is the most confusing," former American Dietetic Association president Nancy Wellman has said, "especially when terms such as '95 percent fat-free' are used." Wellman points out that a turkey frank labeled "80 percent fat-free" actually has 72 percent of its calories from fat.

THE NEW FOOD LABELING

After all the confusion caused by current food labels, won't the new FDA guidelines we've been hearing about come to the rescue and make sense of everything?

The guidelines, which are in the long process of being implemented (and even then, in steps), are, of course, a major step forward. The last sweeping food label changes were made in 1973, when vitamin and mineral contents on labels was the main issue. The new labels could appear on some foods by the middle of 1993, and will be required on all processed foods regulated by the FDA and on all processed meat products regulated by the USDA by May of 1994. Let's take a look at the most significant features of the new food label: the listing of nutrition facts, and the use of standardized descriptive terms.

Nutrition Facts

One of the new label's features will be a revamped nutrition panel, identified by its "Nutrition Facts" heading. Those dietary components that *must* be listed on the panel—and the order in which they must appear—are as follows:

- Total calories
- Calories from fat
- Total fat
- Saturated fat
- Cholesterol
- Sodium
- Total carbohydrate

- Dietary fiber
- Sugars
- Protein
- Vitamin A
- Vitamin C
- Calcium
- Iron

In addition, manufacturers may voluntarily list information about calories from saturated fat, potassium content, and other nutritional components. Interestingly, data on thiamin, riboflavin, and niacin—previously listed on food labels—will no longer be required, as the government has deemed that deficiencies of these vitamins are no longer considered to be of public health significance.

The format for stating the nutrient content per serving has also been revised. For all macronutrients—nutrients needed in relatively large amounts—the amount per serving is listed in grams. In addition, for many of these nutrients, the amount is declared as a percentage of its Daily Value—a recommended daily amount based on a 2,000-calorie diet. Daily Values for the energy producing nutrients are calculated as follows:

- Fat is based on 30 percent of calories.
- Saturated fat is based on 10 percent of calories.
- Carbohydrate is based on 60 percent of calories.
- Protein is based on 10 percent of calories.
- Fiber is based on 11.5 grams of fiber per 1,000 calories.

Because of current public health recommendations, the *maximum* desired number of grams or milligrams of certain nutrients will also be listed for both 2,000- and 2,500-calorie diets. In a 2,000-calorie diet, the suggested amounts of fat and sodium are:

- Total fat: less than 65 grams.

- Saturated fat: less than 20 grams.
- Cholesterol: less than 300 milligrams.
- Sodium: less than 2,400 milligrams.

Further, other nutrients must be listed if they are present in "more than insignificant amounts." Nutrients added to the food must be listed, too.

For clarification, let's take a look at the label shown in Figure 17.1. Here, the total fat is listed as 5 percent of the daily value—in other words, one serving will provide you with 5 percent of the recommended daily intake of that nutrient.

Nutrient Content Descriptions

On the new food label, terms once used as advertising come-ons—and often used misleadingly—now must be applied uniformly to insure that such terms mean the same on each product on which they appear. Following are definitions of some of the most frequently used terms.

- *Free.* The product contains no amount of, or only trivial or "physiologically inconsequential" amounts of, one or more of these components: fat, saturated fat, cholesterol, sodium, sugars, and calories. For instance, "calorie-free" means that there are fewer than 5 calories per serving, and "sugar free" and "fat free" indicate that there are less than 0.5 grams per serving.
- *Low.* This food could be eaten frequently without exceeding dietary guidelines for one or more of the following components: fat, saturated fat, cholesterol, sodium, and calories. Thus, the following terms will be used:

  - *Low fat.* 3 grams or less per serving.
  - *Low saturated fat.* 1 gram or less per serving.
  - *Low sodium.* Less than 140 milligrams per serving.
  - *Very low sodium.* Less than 35 milligrams per serving.

Nutrition Facts

Serving Size ½ cup (114g)
Servings Per Container 4

Amount Per Serving

Calories 90   Calories from Fat 30

	% Daily Value*
Total Fat 3g	5%
Saturated Fat 0g	0%
Cholesterol 0mg	0%
Sodium 300mg	13%
Total Carbohydrate 13g	4%
Dietary Fiber 3g	12%
Sugars 3g	
Protein 3g	

Vitamin A 80% • Vitamin C 60% • Calcium 4% • Iron 4%

*Percent Daily Values are based on
a 2,000 calorie diet. Your Daily
Values may be higher or lower
depending on your calorie needs:

Nutrient		2,000 Calories	2,500 Calories
Total Fat	Less than	65g	80g
Sat Fat	Less than	20g	25g
Cholesterol	Less than	300mg	300mg
Sodium	Less than	2,400mg	2,400mg
Total Carbohydrate		300g	375g
Fiber		25g	30g

Calories per gram:
Fat 9 • Carbohydrates 4 • Protein 4

Figure 17.1 The New Food Label.

- *Low cholesterol.* Less than 20 milligrams per serving.

- *Low calorie.* 40 calories or less per serving.

- *Lean and extra lean.* The following terms can be used to describe the fat content of meat, poultry, seafood, and game meats:

  - *Lean.* Less than 10 grams of fat, less than 4 grams of saturated fat, and less than 95 milligrams of cholesterol per serving and per 100 grams.

  - *Extra lean.* Less than 5 grams of fat, less than 2 grams of saturated fat, and less than 95 milligrams of cholesterol per serving and per 100 grams.

- *High.* One serving of the food contains 20 percent or more of the Daily Value for a particular nutrient.

- *Good source.* One serving of the food contains 10 to 19 percent of the Daily Value for a particular nutrient.

- *Reduced.* A nutritionally altered product contains 25 percent less of a nutrient or of calories than the regular, or reference, product.

- *Less.* A food, whether altered or not, contains 25 percent less of a nutrient or of calories than the reference food.

- *Light.* A nutritionally altered product contains one-third fewer calories or half of the fat of the reference food, *or* the sodium content of a low-calorie, low-fat food has been reduced by 50 percent.

- *More.* One serving of the food, altered or not, contains a nutrient in a quantity that is at least 10 percent of the Daily Value more than the reference food.

A wise consumer would do well to note that manufacturers still have some leeway in the use of these terms—and that "fat free" *still* doesn't always mean that the product contains no fat!

Will New Label Guidelines Help Clear the Confusion?

When the new label laws were first discussed, a number of people cheered them. But, as the FDA and the government opened their ears to an "official comment" period in the beginning of 1992, almost all that was heard was how confusing—and in many ways inadequate—the laws were shaping up to be.

Long before the official comment period, James Tillotson, a Tufts University professor and director at the school's Food Policy Institute, said that he felt there was a danger in telling consumers too much on a label. Tillotson, who held a symposium on the subject, thinks a label should announce calories, carbohydrates, protein, saturated and unsaturated fat, and percentage of calories from fat.

"Other than that," he told the *Chicago Tribune*, "I'm not sure it doesn't become an academic exercise."

Bearing out Tillotson's prediction that confusion may result from the new labeling guidelines, are the first products to hit the markets boasting that they are following the FDA guidelines. As promised, the labels let consumers know, for example, how the product's 13 grams of fat per half-pizza serving stack up to the 65 grams of fat the FDA says is suitable for a healthy consumer. They do the same for saturated fat. This assumes that consumers will be keeping track daily of exactly how many grams of each nutrient they are eating. And, although we're to assume that it wouldn't be smart to go over the referenced amount of fat, what about the 25 grams of fiber listed for a 2,000-calorie diet? Will consumers start making that their cutoff point, too, even though fiber is generally considered to be a good substance that we would be best increasing in our diet?

Also puzzling is the fact that the Daily Values are based on diets of 2,000 or 2,500 calories, *despite* the fact that many people who watch their weight try to consume only about 1,200 per day. How can advice based on this high-calorie consumption be of help to individuals with varying needs?

Another major problem with the new nutrition act that no one seems to be addressing is that nothing in the legislation deals with what is actually in the foods we eat. Many studies have shown that most consumers look at a food label for only about ten seconds before buying a product. (That's why manufacturers make their claims so large and colorful—hoping you won't get to the tiny print regarding ingredients and nutrients and such.) With all the old and new information to appear on labels, there is still absolutely no guarantee that consumers will spend their ten seconds or so reading ingredients.

In any event, it will be quite awhile before all the new labeling regulations—whether they actually prove useful or not—see fruition in our supermarket aisles.

There is already beginning a whole new wave of health hype based on the new labels! Totino's, for example, a frozen pizza made by Pillsbury, sent press kits to daily newspaper food editors boasting of being the first product to use FDA-proposed nutrition labeling information. There was a lot said about how Totino's now has leaner meat and how they are following the new guidelines. There is even a Totino's booklet called *Healthful Hints!* available from the Pillsbury Consumer Center. But there was still no clear word sent with this information on exactly what is in the product. However, anyone who looks at their label in the supermarket knows that, leaner meat or not, there is still a laundry list of ingredients in Totino's, including artificial color and other additives. Since Totino's, which used the new and confusing Daily Reference Values we've been discussing, has indicated how the new guidelines may be presented on labels to the public, it seems we may be in for more—rather than less—confusion.

WHAT YOU CAN DO

Whether you are scrutinizing labels now or looking at new "improved" food labels in the next few years, there are some very simple steps you can take to ensure that you are getting the most nutritious products available. The real key is to trick the labels, rather than letting them trick you. How can you trick the labels? Just don't read them.

Don't read labels? Well, for the most part. Ignore all claims, and read only two parts of the label: The ingredients listing and the nutritional information per serving. This information is on current nutrition labels and will also be on those that result from the new nutrition act.

Instead of looking at those "cholesterol-free" or other colorful banners (not to mention contests, giveaways, and so on) on the front, take just ten seconds or so to flip the package around and read the fine print. Believe it or not, this will give you all the information most informed shoppers need to reduce drastically their intake of enriched products, refined sugar, additives, chemicals, and preservatives.

This may seem obvious and logical, but I am constantly surprised that most people giving mainstream nutritional advice never suggest it.

For example, in the beginning of 1990, a major publisher announced with much fanfare a first-of-its-kind book, compiled by a respected registered dietitian. It promised "nutritional information" for all "lite" and other modified foods on the market. Lots of products are listed, broken down in every imaginable way, but—to my and undoubtedly many a reader's surprise—no ingredient is listed anywhere.

Similarly, as a food editor, I recently was sent samples of a column from a major syndicate, along with its sales pitch. The column, written by a dietitian, was touted as being *the* place where readers could find all pertinent information regarding food labels. The author even compared and rated products head-to-head. Again, however, ingredient listings were not a part of her nutritional criteria. Make them, no matter what, a part of yours, and you can't help but be healthier.

18

Vitamins and Minerals

Many doctors say that people who eat a balanced, varied diet do not need vitamin supplementation. However, with the abundance of overprocessed, nutrient-deficient foods in this country, as well as the enormous number of people who are undereating—three out of five women and one out of five men at any given time are dieting—no one, but no one, seems to be able to find where most of the people eating the varied, balanced diets are hiding.

Although many in the medical community still chant what is quickly becoming an outdated statement—"You can get all the nutrients you need from a balanced diet"—most people in the United States simply are not eating a balanced diet.

For example, studies have shown that many people do not eat even one serving of fruits or vegetables a day. A United States Department of Agriculture survey of 21,000 people found that not one of them got the recommended daily allowance (RDA, which is the absolute minimum advised) of any of ten nutrients needed for basic good health. Those people were low in iron, folacin (folic acid), calcium, zinc, water, fiber, beta-carotene, vitamin B₆, vitamin C, and magnesium.

In fact, according to an analysis by Annemarie Crocetti, M.D., and Helen Guthrie, Ph.D., in "Eating Behavior and Associated Nutrient Quality of Diets," which is part of the *USDA Food Con-*

sumption Survey, 97 percent of the United States population does not eat a balanced diet. The survey found the population in general had significant shortages of these vitamins and minerals: A, B₁, B₂, B₆, B₁₂, C, niacin, calcium, iron, and magnesium.

Many of us, of course, are aware that we may not be getting all the vitamins and minerals we need from the foods we choose. Forty percent of all adults and an even higher percentage of children take vitamin supplements daily. In the process, they have created an industry that, according to the Center for Vitamin and Mineral Communications, in 1992 surpassed the $6 billion mark.

However, as in so many areas of health where we have taken matters into our own hands, many people who pop those vitamin pills into their mouths readily admit that they are not sure about the difference between vitamins and minerals or of what they do inside our bodies. First, let's take a look at some of the basics when it comes to vitamins and minerals. Then we can study the RDAs and why they simply may not be doing you nutritional justice.

WHAT ARE VITAMINS AND MINERALS?

If you are eating a natural diet full of vitamins and minerals and if you are taking a vitamin/mineral supplement, then after reading about all the important functions of vitamins and minerals, I think you'll give yourself a pat on the on the back.

Vitamins are organic compounds, and minerals are inorganic elements. They are essential for proper growth and development. Human beings cannot live without them. Each vitamin or mineral performs a specific function in the body. For example, vitamin A is essential for normal growth and vision, as well as healthy skin, teeth, gums, and hair. Many studies have also shown a link between adequate vitamin A intake and cancer prevention.

Vitamins and minerals are nutrients. They are also called "micronutrients" because, although essential, compared with other nutrients such as water, fat, carbohydrates, and proteins, human beings need them in small amounts. However, as we've seen by the surveys that have been undertaken, many people do not even get the small amounts of vitamins and minerals that are necessary.

Vitamins cannot be produced by the body and must be provided through the diet or by supplementation. However, once consumed and absorbed, vitamins and minerals become part of the body structure. They stay in the body for varied amounts of time and work with the blood, bones, muscles, and cells.

Water-soluble vitamins stay in the body for only a short period of time. The B vitamins and vitamin C are water-soluble. Fat-soluble vitamins stay in the body longer, which is why you have to be careful not to take large doses in the form of supplements. Such vitamins are stored in the body's fat tissues and organs. Vitamins A, D, E, and K are fat-soluble.

Minerals come in the micro or macro varieties. Microminerals are also referred to as trace minerals. Although essential, they are needed in only small amounts. Microminerals include chromium, copper, iodine, iron, manganese, potassium, selenium, and zinc. Macrominerals are needed in larger amounts. They include calcium, magnesium, and phosphorus. Minerals are stored in bones, muscles and other parts of the body.

IF WE FOLLOW THE RDAS, WHY WOULD WE NEED SUPPLEMENTATION?

As we've seen from governmental and other studies, almost no one in the United States is even getting the recommended daily allowances (RDAs) of vitamins, minerals, and other essential nutrients.

But let's say, just for speculation, that some of us—especially readers of this book, who obviously care about their health—are straight-A "RDA-ers." In other words, let's assume we are getting 100 percent of the RDAs.

Unfortunately, even if you are a person who safeguards your health and is valiantly trying to prevent yourself from becoming the prey of major diseases, this "100 percent" might not be enough.

The RDAs are established by the Food and Nutrition Board of the National Academy of Sciences' National Research Council. The first RDAs were published in 1941, and new editions are published about every five years. Although much of the public seems to think the RDAs are an ideal to shoot for, the numbers were actually established as nutritional *minimums* to ensure against diseases like scurvy, which can lay its claim when people are severely malnourished. But what about people who do not simply want to avoid the most severe cases of malnutrition, but who want to glow with health and vitality? The RDAs do nothing to answer such a question.

Current food labels contain U.S. RDAs, a simplified version of RDAs. When you scan food labels, you will see no special notes or clarifications, but literature from the Committee on Dietary Allowances of the Food and Nutrition Board—the creator of the RDAs—makes no bones about how minimal the RDAs are.

The committee's literature states, "For certain nutrients the requirements may be assessed as the amount that will just prevent failure of a specific function or the development of specific deficiency signs—an amount that may differ greatly from that required to maintain maximum body stores. Thus, there are differences of opinion about the criteria that should be used to establish requirements."

The committee also points out that all RDAs were developed only for healthy people. They admit, in their literature, that "healthy" is a murky term. Also, they write that the RDAs are not meant in any way to cover anyone who is not healthy. Many scientists and researchers argue that there are very few truly healthy people left in our society, what with the ravages of heart disease, cancer, and diseases like hypertension, arthritis, and osteoporosis. They say much of our population is, in fact, chronically ill and would not be covered by the RDAs for healthy individuals.

Also not listed on the product labels you peruse is the number of calories on which the RDAs are based. The RDAs assume that the average woman is eating a diet of about 2,000 calories per day and the average man about 3,000 calories. Many people, of course—especially in this age of dieting for weight control—consume fewer calories.

A small remaining part of the medical establishment remarks, "You don't need supplementation if you eat a varied, balanced diet," but even those members nearly all concede that there are groups to which this advice does not apply. Supplementation is necessary in many cases, they say, for women who are pregnant or breast-feeding, women with heavy menstrual periods, vegetarians, and people on medication.

VITAMINS AND MINERALS AS A MEANS OF DISEASE PREVENTION

Besides the fact that the RDAs are only the minimum amounts of vitamins and minerals needed to avoid malnutrition, the calculations that have gone into determining them do not even take into account all the exciting research in recent years that has shown certain vitamins and minerals possibly playing a vital role in disease prevention. Why would we want to ignore this kind of information when deciding what food or supplementation choices to make?

Following are just a few examples of some of this important recent research:

- In March 1992, news services reported that researchers had found more evidence linking vitamin A and vitamin C with a lowered risk of cancer. Vitamin A was shown to possibly reduce the risk of lung, esophageal, and bladder cancers. New studies on vitamin C showed that it appears to protect against esophageal and gastric cancers.

- A 1988 Finnish study of 21,170 men showed that vitamin E appeared to lower cancer risk in young men and non-smokers.

- 1990 research out of the University of Mississippi School of Pharmacy showed that vitamins C and E may protect against heart disease. Dr. Anthony Verlangieri, who led the study, said those vitamins seemed to reverse arterial damage brought on by high-fat diets. High but safe doses of vitamins C and E slowed the progression of arterial damage, and thus heart disease, by 50 percent in test monkeys. The vitamins also caused a 30-percent healing of arterial damage. As a result of his studies, Verlangieri takes 1,000 to 2,000 milligrams of vitamin C and 200 to 400 international units (IUs) of vitamin E daily. Scientists say his research helps explain why eating a lot of fruits and vegetables—rich in vitamin C—has been shown to cut heart disease risk.

- Niacin, a vitamin with drug-like action, can cut cholesterol, reports the Mayo Clinic and countless other research centers. Daily doses of one-half gram to six grams of niacin decrease the levels of overall and LDL (bad) cholesterol, increase the levels of HDL (good) cholesterol, and lower the levels of triglycerides (blood fat), according to Mayo. Be sure, though, to check with your physician regarding what might be the best dosage for you.

- Cancer. Heart disease. High cholesterol. These are all major health issues. But what about the countless little improvements that might come with getting enough vitamins and minerals? A 1990 study from the U.S. Department of Agriculture shed light on just such an issue.

  The study showed that small amounts of the nutrient boron could make a difference in women's lives. Researchers discovered that when a woman's boron intake is very low (about one-quarter milligram or less per day), her motor performance suffers. Brain waves change, and alertness drops. When the women's diets contained little boron, they couldn't tap their fingers as fast, follow a target as accurately, or respond as quickly when solving a puzzle. (Men would probably have similar reactions.) Three milligrams of boron are considered adequate by the researchers—although many people, because they don't eat enough fruits and vegetables, do not ingest that much. Boron is most abundant in apples, grapes, pears, broccoli, and carrots. You might just wonder, if it's robbing you of your alertness or your ability to solve a puzzle, then what other little areas in your life might be deficient because of a seemingly minor vitamin or mineral deficiency?

WHAT DOSAGE OF VITAMINS AND MINERALS SHOULD I TAKE?

As most health professionals state, it is important to get as many vitamins and minerals as possible from the foods you eat. If you follow the natural, nutrient-packed suggestions throughout this book, you should already be way ahead of the game—and when you take in vitamins and minerals in your foods, you are also getting the fiber that goes along with the food.

However, almost no one gets even the minimal RDA of vitamins and minerals from their food, so you should probably take a vitamin and mineral supplement that supplies 100 percent of the RDAs for most vitamins and minerals and even higher amounts of such key vitamins as A, C, and E. Such a supplement, along with your attempt at eating a fruit- and vegetable-filled, disease-preventing diet, would probably ensure that you are getting quite a quality variety of vitamins and minerals.

An important thing to keep in mind when purchasing supplements is to use the same judgment you would when buying healthful food. Some supplements contain sugar, fillers, and artificial colors. You don't need those things in your food, let alone in your vitamin supplement! Supplement labels, like food labels, list ingredients. Look for labels that state the pills contain no sugar, artificial additives, or other such ingredients.

OPTIMAL DAILY REQUIREMENTS

Some people, however, may want to take all this information one step further and make even more of a commitment to supplementation for possible major disease prevention. Shari Lieberman, a Ph.D. candidate and registered dietitian with a master's degree in clinical nutrition, has developed what she calls ODAs, or Optimal Daily Allowances.

The ODAs were created, according to Lieberman, because "we are not meeting the RDAs even if we are eating the 'perfect' diet. The foods available to us do not contain the amounts of vitamins and minerals they should contain, including loss of nutrients through shipping, storage, and processing. We require higher levels of vitamins and minerals owing to the constant bombardment of stress factors in our environment such as pollution and emotional stress. And vitamins and minerals are never 100-percent absorbed."

Unlike many health professionals, Lieberman, when creating her supplement recommendations, took into account all the latest research on immunity enhancement and on preventing cardiovascular disease, cancer, diabetes, and other disorders. Table 18.1 provides a quick reference to the functions and sources of the vitamins and minerals that we all need, as well as each nutrient's RDA and ODA. The basic ODAs, indicated by the range presented in the table, will provide many people with optimum general physical and mental health. However, if there are factors in your life that place you at a higher risk for certain diseases—for instance, if you have a family history of heart disease—you may want to increase the amount of the appropriate supplement. Please note that for some nutrients—boron, for example—RDAs and ODAs have not yet been determined. For these nutrients, a recommended range has been indicated, followed by an asterisk (*), which indicates that this dosage is not an ODA. Naturally, before beginning any supplement program, it's wise to consult a qualified health professional.

When it comes to supplementation, whether you start with one multivitamin or leap into a full Optimal Daily Requirement regimen, you may well be ensuring a healthier future for yourself. Certainly, eating a healthy diet is essential. But supplementation can provide the extra nutritional insurance you need to feel your best.

Table 18.1. Quick-Reference Nutrient Guide

Nutrient	Major Uses	Food Sources	RDA	ODA
Vitamin A; beta-carotene	Prevents night blindness and other eye problems. May be useful for acne and other skin disorders Enhances immunity. Cancer prevention. May heal gastrointestinal ulcers. Protects against pollution. Needed for epithelial tissue maintenance and repair.	Fish liver oils, animal livers, green and yellow fruits and vegetables	4,000– 5,000 IU	10,000–75,000 IU (in a mixture of A and beta-carotene)
Vitamin D	Required for calcium and phosphorus absorption and utilization. Prevention and treatment of osteoporosis. Enhances immunity.	Fish liver oils, fatty saltwater fish. Vitamin D-fortified dairy products, eggs	400 IU	400–600 IU

*From *The Real Vitamin & Mineral Book* by Shari Lieberman and Nancy Bruning. Garden City Park, NY: Avery Publishing Group, 1990.

Nutrient	Major Uses	Food Sources	RDA	ODA
Vitamin E	Antioxidant. Cancer prevention. Cardiovascular disease prevention. Improves circulation. Tissue repair. May prevent age spots. Useful in treating fibrocystic breasts. Useful in treating PMS.	Cold-pressed vegetable oils, whole grains, dark-green leafy vegetables, nuts, legumes	8–10 IU	200–800 IU
Vitamin K	Needed for blood clotting. May play a role in bone formation. May prevent osteoporosis.	Green leafy vegetables	65–80 mcg	
B Complex B-1 (thiamin); B-2 (riboflavin); B-3 (niacin, niacinamide) B-6 (pyridoxine)	Maintains healthy nerves, skin, eyes, hair, liver, mouth, muscle tone in gastrointestinal tract. B vitamins are coenzymes involved in energy production. Emotional or physical stress increases need. May be useful for depression or anxiety.	Unrefined whole grains, liver, green leafy vegetables, fish, poultry, eggs, meat, nuts, beans	1.2–14 mg	25–300 mg

B-1: High-carbohydrate diet increases need.
B-2: May be useful with B-6 for treatment of carpal tunnel syndrome. May prevent cataracts. Increased need with oral contraceptives. Increased need with strenuous exercise.
B-3: Useful for circulatory problems. Lowers serum cholesterol and triglycerides.
B-6: May be useful in preventing oxalate stones. May be used as mild diuretic. May be useful for PMS. Increased need with oral contraceptives. May be useful in treating asthma.

Nutrient	Major Uses	Food Sources	RDA	ODA
B-12 (cobalamin)	Needed for fat and carbohydrate metabolism. Prevention and treatment of B-12 anemia. Maintains proper nervous system function. May be useful for anxiety and depression.	Kidney, liver, egg, herring, mackerel, milk, cheese, tofu, seafood	2 mcg	25–300 mcg

Nutrient	Major Uses	Food Sources	RDA	ODA
Folic acid	Works closely with B-12. Involved in protein metabolism. Needed for healthy cell division and replication. Prevention and treatment of folic acid anemia. Stress may increase need. May be useful for depression and anxiety. May be useful in treating cervical dysplasia. Oral contraceptives may increase need.	Beef, lamb, pork, chicken liver, green leafy vegetables, whole wheat, bran, yeast	180–200 mcg	400–1,200 mcg
Pantothenic acid	Needed in fat, protein, and carbohydrate metabolism. Needed for synthesis of hormones and cholesterol. Needed for red blood cell production. Needed for nerve transmission. Vital for healthy function of the adrenal glands. May be useful for joint inflammation. May be useful for depression and anxiety.	Eggs, salt-water fish, pork, beef, milk, whole wheat, beans, fresh vegetables	None	25–300 mg
Biotin	Needed for metabolism of protein, fats, and carbohydrates. Not enough data available, but deficiencies may be implicated in high serum cholesterol, seborrheic dermatitis, and certain nervous system disorders.	Meat, cooked egg yolk, poultry, yeast, soybeans, milk, saltwater fish, whole grains	None	25–300 mcg
Choline and Inositol	Involved in metabolism of fat and cholesterol and absorption and utilization of fat. Choline makes an important brain neurotransmitter.	Egg yolk, whole grains, vegetables, organ meats, fruits, milk	None	25–300 mg

Nutrient	Major Uses	Food Sources	RDA	ODA
PABA	Needed for protein metabolism. Needed for folic acid metabolism. Used topically as a sunscreen.	Liver, kidney, whole grains, molasses	None	25–300 mg

A combination of all the B vitamins can usually be found in B-complex and multivitamin formulas. If you wish to take any additional B vitamins, please make sure you are taking a complete B complex first.

Nutrient	Major Uses	Food Sources	RDA	ODA
Vitamin C (ascorbic acid)	Growth and repair of tissues. May reduce cholesterol. Antioxidant. Cancer prevention. Enhances immunity. Stress increases requirement. May reduce high blood pressure. May prevent atherosclerosis. Protects against pollution.	Green vegetables, berries, citrus fruit	60 mg	500–5,000 mg (higher during stress or illness)
Calcium	Needed for healthy bones and teeth. Needed for nerve transmission. Used for muscle function. May lower blood pressure. Osteoporosis prevention.	Dairy foods, salmon, sardines, green leafy vegetables, seafood	1,200 mg	1,000–1,500 mg
Phosphorus	Necessary for healthy bones. Needed for production of energy. Used as a buffering agent. Needed for utilization of protein, fats, and carbohydrates.	Available in most foods; sodas can be very high	800 mg	Generally available through foods: 200–400 mg
Magnesium	Needed for healthy bones. Involved in nerve transmission. Needed for muscle function. Used in energy formation. Needed for healthy blood vessels. May lower blood pressure.	Widely distributed in foods, especially dairy foods, meat, fish, seafood	280–350 mg	500–700 mg

Nutrient	Major Uses	Food Sources	RDA	ODA
Zinc	Needed for wound healing. Maintains taste and smell acuity. Needed for healthy immune system. Protects liver from chemical damage.	Oysters, fish, seafood, meats, poultry, whole grains, legumes	12–15 mg	22.5–50 mg
Iron	Vital for blood formation. Needed for energy production. Required for healthy immune system.	Meat, poultry, fish, liver, eggs, green leafy vegetables, whole grain or enriched breads and cereals	10–15 mg	15–30 mg
Copper	Involved in blood formation. Needed for healthy nerves. Needed for taste sensitivity. Used in energy production. Needed for healthy bone development.	Widely distributed in foods, copper cookware, and copper plumbing	None	Needs can generally be met through food: 0.5–2 mg
Manganese	Needed for protein and fat metabolism. Used in energy formation. Required for normal bone growth and reproduction. Needed for healthy nerves. Needed for healthy blood sugar regulation. Needed for healthy immune system.	Nuts, seeds, whole grains, avocado, seaweed	None	15–30 mg
Chromium	Required for glucose metabolism. May prevent diabetes. May reduce cholesterol.	Brewer's yeast, beer, meat, cheese, whole grains	None	200–600 mcg
Selenium	Cancer prevention. Heart disease prevention.	Depends on soil content, may be in grains and meat	55–70 mcg	50–400 mcg (50–100 mcg for those who live in high-selenium areas)

Nutrient	Major Uses	Food Sources	RDA	ODA
Iodine	Needed for healthy thyroid gland. Prevents goiter.	Iodized salts, seafood, saltwater fish, kelp	150 mcg	50–300 mcg (50–150 mcg for those who use iodized salt)
Potassium	May lower blood pressure. Needed for energy storage. Needed for nerve transmission, muscle contraction, and hormone secretion.	Dairy foods, meat, poultry, fish, fruit, legumes, whole grains, vegetables	None	99–300 mg
Boron	Prevents bone loss. May enhance bone density.	Fruits, vegetables	None	3–6 mg*
EPA	Prevents heart disease. May lower blood pressure. May lower triglycerides. May lower cholesterol. Prevents excess blood clotting. May relieve inflammatory and allergic reactions. May inhibit cancer. May enhance immune system.	Cold-water fish	None	250–3,000 mg*
GLA	May prevent heart disease. Relieves allergic reactions. Relieves eczema. Relieves arthritis. Relieves PMS symptoms. May assist in weight loss.	Evening primrose, borage, black currant oils	None	70–240 mg*
Garlic	May lower blood pressure. May enhance immune system. May prevent heart disease. May lower triglycerides. May lower cholesterol. Antibacterial, antiviral, antifungal. Prevents excess blood clotting. May prevent cancer.	Garlic	None	200–1,200 mg*

Nutrient	Major Uses	Food Sources	RDA	ODA
Coenzyme Q-10 (CoQ)	Cell energy and metabolism. Prevents cell damage. May be useful in heart disease such as angina, congestive heart failure, arrhythmia, high blood pressure. May protect heart muscle and promote faster recovery from heart attack and heart surgery.	None	None	10–300 mg*
Germanium	Needed for cell metabolism. May prevent or slow growth of cancer. May enhance immune system. May lower blood pressure. Relieves pain.	A variety of medicinal plants	None	30–150 mg*

19

Caffeine

A southern truck driver got a lot more than he bargained for when he upped his intake of caffeinated cola from ten cans a day to twenty. Instead of being more alert for his all-night treks, the driver found his next destination to be a mental hospital.

The driver, who was one of the subjects in a study conducted by psychiatrist Andrew Mebane of the Ochsner Clinic in New Orleans, began acting so strangely after he increased his caffeine intake that he was diagnosed with schizophrenia, a mental illness characterized by disordered thinking, hallucinations, and delusions. However, when doctors realized caffeine might be the culprit, and the man stopped drinking beverages that contain it, all his symptoms disappeared.

Some researchers might say the man was lucky to have made that unplanned pit stop in the mental ward. Perhaps, they might say, his abrupt change of habit will preclude him from suffering from some of these other problems shown to have possible links to consistent caffeine use: Hypertension, coronary heart disease and heart attack risk, high cholesterol, brittle bones, certain kinds of cancer, infertility, and (for women) breast lumps and aggravation of the symptoms of premenstrual syndrome.

More than 80 percent of the population in the United States is thought to partake regularly of beverages and foods that contain caffeine. But the public's interest in nutrition and health has mushroomed in recent years, and many people are cutting caffeine from their diet or seriously thinking about doing so. More and more products cater to this growing crowd by boasting that they contain no caffeine. However, just as with many of the other substances discussed in this book, many of those same people readily admit they are unsure about what caffeine does when it enters their body or precisely why they might want to avoid it.

First, let's take a look at just what caffeine is and what it does once it enters your system. Then we can examine what the scientific community has said about the subject.

WHAT IS CAFFEINE?

Methylxanthines are a group of compounds found in more than fifty types of plants. Caffeine is a methylxanthine. It is also a drug, classified pharmacologically as a mild stimulant. It stimulates the central nervous system. Is that what *you* think about when you grab for a sip of diet soda or a swig of coffee? Our Stone Age ancestors probably didn't think about such things, either. But caffeine use has been documented as far back as the Stone Age.

Caffeine is present in coffee, tea, cola, and chocolate. Many people get used to the "up"—the stimulant effect—they think they feel after drinking beverages that contain caffeine. Others know that if they partake of a caffeine-containing beverage in the evening, they might have trouble sleeping or, in fact, be up all night.

But what is really happening inside the body to cause such effects? In addition to stimulating the central nervous system, caffeine can increase heartbeat and metabolic rate. It can also step up the production of stomach acid and dilate blood vessels.

Although many caffeine users are unaware of exactly what the drug is doing inside their body, most believe its effects wear off fairly quickly. However, according to a recent scientific status summary from the Institute of Food Technologists' Expert Panel on Food Safety and Nutrition, the half-life of caffeine can last several days. A half-life is the time it takes the body to eliminate only half of a substance that has been introduced into it. The report goes on to say that factors such as smoking, age, sex, and hormonal conditions can all come into play in determining how long it takes for the effects of caffeine to dissipate.

IS CAFFEINE SAFE?

Caffeine is one of more than 3,000 food additives we use. It also occurs naturally in substances such as coffee beans and cocoa. If our government has approved it and it's been used for years, many people assume it must be safe. But is it?

Caffeine and many other substances have been labeled "Generally Regarded as Safe" (GRAS) by the FDA. But even when the government labels something as GRAS, it often notes that further testing is still needed. Look in any food additive dictionary or reference guide and you will see plenty of additives—including caffeine—that bear the further-testing-is-needed stamp. However, when we scan a packaged food's ingredient list, we receive no such information.

The FDA also states that absolutely no additive is ever granted permanent approval. The agency makes the caveat that any additive can be pulled at any time, either permanently or for further review.

What is especially interesting about caffeine and so many other additives is that before they were given GRAS status they were not required to have been tested at all. It is important for any health-concerned consumer to be aware of the Food Additives Amendment, which was added in 1958 to the United States Federal Food, Drug, and Cosmetics Act. The amendment simply said that all additives in use before 1958—which included caffeine—could be considered GRAS.

Additives were allowed to be GRAS simply because there was no evidence yet that they might be a health danger. As so many of us now know, however, it takes many years for certain health problems to become evident. And with diseases like cancer, it's often impossible to know what caused them.

CAFFEINE STUDIES

Caffeine was finally reviewed at the request of the FDA in 1978—twenty years after the passage of the Food Additives Amendment.

Caffeine was left on the GRAS list, but the reviewers did note that additional research should be done.

The report to the FDA stated, "While no evidence in the available information on caffeine demonstrates a hazard to the public when it is used in cola-type beverages at levels that are now current and in the manner now practiced, uncertainties exist requiring that additional studies be conducted."

It is important to note that those conducting the research for the government did so only on caffeine as an additive and not on the naturally occurring caffeine in coffee or tea.

Even without further research, problems stemming from caffeine use had already been given a name—caffeinism—by the scientific community. Lay people often refer to this as "coffee nerves," but scientists have determined a number of other symptoms. You might not even recognize these as being related to the use of caffeine: Anxiety, insomnia, diarrhea, heart palpitations, malabsorption of iron, and headaches.

Let's take a look at some of the things you are not going to read about on a coffee package label or a can of soda. Independent scientists reviewing caffeine on their own, rather than for the government, have found from testing caffeine and coffee over the years a number of areas of concern: Cardiovascular disease, birth defects, infertility, brittle bones, high blood pressure, premenstrual syndrome, ulcers, bladder cancer, pancreatic cancer, and addiction.

As early as 1972, a study of 13,000 patients showed a link between coffee drinking and heart attack. A study a year later confirmed the findings. Since then, some studies have not shown the link, while others (including a recent one of 129,000 people) have reconfirmed it. At the least, some questions still exist.

Certain statements in the media show just how ambiguous this kind of information can be. A 1989 issue of the respected health magazine *Hippocrates* (now renamed *Health*) stated, "The experts now say that most people who drink a few cups of coffee each day have little to worry about. . . . Still a few health worries linger, especially for pregnant women and people at risk for heart disease." We've already shown how prevalent heart disease is. It is the country's top killer. Millions of people are affected. Most have no idea they are at risk. The first warning sign for most people is the actual heart attack. If those are the people who should be avoiding caffeine, they often have no way of identifying themselves.

The studies that have linked caffeine and coffee use to heart attack risk are concerned mainly with the fact that coffee has been shown to increase cholesterol. I think the logic behind some of the ways the newest data is being interpreted is, in a word, scary.

For example, "Coffee doesn't increase risk of heart disease" was the optimistic headline over a February 1992 *USA Today* story. The study being reported on was done by a physician at Kaiser Permanente Medical Center in Kensington, Maryland, and was published in the *New England Journal of Medicine*. One hundred healthy men were studied. These were the facts: The men were taken off all caffeine and their cholesterol levels dropped. Some of the men then drank four cups of coffee a day. Levels of LDL (bad) cholesterol increased by six points and raised the heart disease risk by 9 percent! Levels of HDL (good) cholesterol increased three points. So, therefore, although coffee raised the men's total cholesterol number, the reporters figured that the slight increase in good cholesterol might cancel the risk! But if you saw such a positive headline about coffee use, wouldn't you think it meant that the bad cholesterol had *decreased*? Instead, it *increased*, and the logic employed tried to make us believe that was good news!

The Surgeon General and National Academy of Sciences recommend not drinking coffee when pregnant. Although some studies have not confirmed it, the studies on which the government based its opinion showed that birth defects were found in the offspring of 20 percent of rats who were force-fed caffeine while pregnant. Higher percentages of miscarriages have sometimes been noted in human populations where caffeine intake was high. Stillbirths and infants with low birth weights have also resulted.

A recent study was the first and only one to consider the link between caffeine intake and fertility. It showed that women who drank more than one cup of coffee per day were only 50 percent as likely to conceive as those who drank less.

"Caffeine makes its way into all parts of the reproductive tract," the study's leader, epidemiologist Allen Wilcox of the National Institute of Environmental Health Sciences, told a health journal. "We can't say how it affects [reproduction], but it's in the vicinity of where the action is."

A 1990 study done jointly by scientists at Boston University and Brown University showed that people who drank a lot of coffee, tea, or caffeinated cola were much more apt to develop osteoporosis and have life-threatening bone breaks as senior citizens.

The findings showed that people who drank between two and a half and three cups of coffee or tea, or more than a few cans of cola, per day were 69 percent more likely to develop osteoporosis.

A 1991 Stanford University study showed that healthy men who drank three to six cups of coffee a day experienced a significant drop in blood pressure when they stopped drinking coffee.

The Stanford researchers said many of the previous studies that found coffee having no effect on blood pressure contained too few patients and thus should be discarded. The Stanford study included 120 men.

Oregon State University studied almost 900 women in 1990 and found that the intake of drinks containing caffeine aggravated symptoms of premenstrual syndrome (PMS). This study offers the most specific data to date connecting PMS symptoms to caffeine, although researchers have suspected the link since the early 1980s.

Until recently, PMS, which may affect nearly three out of four women at some point in their lives, was thought to be a psychological problem. However, even women who drank just one glass of a caffeine-containing beverage a day were shown to be more likely to have PMS than those who did not.

Since caffeine increases stomach acid, it has been shown, at the least, to aggravate existing ulcers. Some scientists believe beverages containing caffeine can also play a role in the development of ulcers.

Some studies over the years have shown links between caffeine consumption and bladder cancer, pancreatic cancer, and fibrocystic breast disease, although other studies have failed to find such connections.

Finally, if all of the other possible health concerns are not enough, caffeine is addictive. Some experts believe that if caffeine were an additive first coming to our attention today, it would not be allowed in our foods and beverages. Dr. Jere E. Goyan, a top physician with the FDA, was quoted in 1991 by the Associated Press as saying, "If caffeine were up for approval today, it probably could only be obtained by prescription."

ELIMINATING CAFFEINE
AND THE DECAFFEINATION QUESTION

If thoughts of cardiovascular disease, high blood pressure, birth defects, or osteoporosis give you pause when you lift your morning coffee or sip a diet soda with your lunch, you are not alone. Plenty of people have kicked the caffeine habit.

However, since caffeine is addictive, you can expect some withdrawal symptoms. The most notable of these is usually a gradually subsiding headache that may persist for three or four days.

If you don't want to quit caffeine cold turkey, the American Dietetic Association offers the following tips:

- Drink instant coffee (or the new "light" coffee, which has half the caffeine) for a while before totally giving up caffeine. A cup of regular instant coffee generally contains less caffeine than a cup of regular brewed coffee.

- Drink a mixture of half regular and half decaffeinated coffee.

- Brew tea for less time. A one-minute brewing, versus a three-minute brewing, can cut caffeine in half.

Once you are off caffeine, you may, like many people, turn to decaffeinated coffee. However, recently there has been much in the media about the health effects of decaffeinated coffee—a beverage that many ex-caffeine junkies hailed.

The questions raised concern the method used for decaffeination. Like many health issues, this is probably one many of us never before thought about when we drank our decaf. Well, that cup of decaf may have gotten that way through a chemical method or by another method that uses water as a buffer. Decaffeinating agents can include pretreated charcoal, oils extracted from coffee beans, carbon dioxide, ethyl acetate, and methylene chloride.

Methylene chloride has been the chief culprit in critics' concern over decaffeination. The FDA banned the use of the chemical in aerosol cosmetic products when test animals developed tumors after inhaling the gas. The FDA has not banned the use of the gas in decaffeination, because the residue left is thought to be minimal. However, consumer concern has caused many coffee processors to switch to other methods. But even with the water method, the water is often exposed to methylene chloride and other chemicals. Just another thing to be aware of when you are reading those coffee can labels in the supermarket!

20

MSG

Carl Jillian, a banker in Minneapolis, didn't realize there was something fishy about his tuna fish. In an effort to eat a low-fat diet, Jillian brought a tuna fish salad to work for lunch three or four times a week. In addition to eating a low-fat diet, Jillian had eliminated caffeine, refined sugar, and monosodium glutamate (MSG) from his diet. Or had he?

The brand of tuna fish Jillian ate—like many other tuna brands—included hydrolyzed protein as an ingredient. Hydrolyzed protein, however, as well as a number of other ingredients regularly added to foods, includes MSG. In fact, Jillian could have actually been getting a triple dose of MSG in a product labeled "No MSG added" because the tuna also contained "natural flavorings" and "vegetable broth"—types of ingredients that often include MSG.

Although many health-conscious people readily admit to trying to avoid MSG, many are just as ready to admit they are unsure about exactly what MSG is or why they're avoiding it. Therefore, before we look into the virtual laundry list of ingredients MSG may be hiding within, and at why you may want to avoid them, let's take a look at what MSG is and what scientists have discovered it does to you once you ingest it.

WHAT IS MSG?

MSG is the salt of glutamatic acid, one of the twenty amino acids that make up proteins. Glutamate found naturally in foods produces a distinctive flavor. Foods with a high natural glutamate content include tomatoes, mushrooms, and Parmesan cheese. By chemically producing monosodium glutamate, food manufacturers try to achieve that same flavor-enhancing effect.

Monosodium glutamate—and other ingredients that contain it—is added to hundreds of processed foods. The production of MSG is a multibillion-dollar business, according to investigative research by Dr. George Schwartz, a physician and medical textbook author who wrote *In Bad Taste: The MSG Syndrome*, a 1988 book that so far is the only one devoted solely to MSG.

According to the MSG industry, the United States per capita consumption of MSG increased by at least 30 percent between 1982 and 1992. That means the average American now consumes about half a pound of MSG per year. American companies add 45 million pounds of hydrolyzed proteins to their products each year, according to the International Hydrolyzed Protein Council, a trade group in Washington, D.C. Hydrolyzed proteins always contain MSG, in amounts up to 50 percent.

MSG has been added to foods in the United States for over eighty years. In the Orient, the substance has a centuries-long history. Although the Western scientific community generally agrees that taste comprises four components—sweet, sour, salty, and bitter—Japanese scientists believe a fifth component is *umami*, the taste in MSG associated with protein.

THE CHINESE RESTAURANT SYNDROME

MSG is in a huge array of foods, from fast foods to canned soups to—as mentioned earlier—tuna fish. However, the first time much of the public heard about MSG was in association with a condition called the Chinese restaurant syndrome.

The term was coined to describe symptoms some people believe they experience after eating Chinese food. An exchange of letters in a 1968 edition of the *New England Journal of Medicine* between Dr. Ho Man Kwok, a Maryland physician, and other physician readers of the periodical was the first major exposure given to the syndrome. Kwok wrote about symptoms he experienced after eating at Chinese restaurants. He described a numbness at the base of his neck, as well as in his arms and back, after eating Chinese food. Kwok and other doctors stated they believed that the MSG used so prevalently in Chinese restaurant food was the culprit behind such symptoms. Since 1968, tens of thousands of people have reported feeling the effects of the Chinese restaurant syndrome. Many restaurants now prominently display signs saying that they no longer add MSG to food, and others are happy to accept orders that include a request that the additive not be used.

The Glutamate Association of the United States, a powerful Atlanta-based trade group, explains the Chinese restaurant syndrome by stating that its effects may be due to other elements often found in Chinese food, such as a high sodium or histamine content. They also state that certain vegetables used in the cuisine might be causing the effect.

The Glutamate Association also points to the fact that an average Chinese meal has no more glutamate than an average Italian meal. This, they say, is because Italian cuisine relies heavily on tomatoes, mushrooms, and Parmesan cheese—all natural sources of glutamate. However, Schwartz and other MSG researchers argue that there is a very significant difference between the way the body reacts to natural glutamate and the way it reacts to chemically derived MSG. We'll take a closer look at that in a moment.

Along with the sharp increase in the addition of MSG—in outright and hidden forms—to thousands of processed foods in recent years, there has been an increase in the reports of symptoms people feel they have experienced after ingesting the additive. A flushed face, tingling, and burning sensations have been reported as symptoms. Headaches, irritability, cramps, and diarrhea are also common complaints. In some people, asthma is triggered.

SCIENTISTS LOOK AT MSG

Scientists estimate that anywhere from 1 to 30 percent of the population may have some sensitivity to MSG, and a number of those who believe they are sensitive have stepped forward and reported their symptoms. In many areas of science, anecdotal evidence (personal experience) is disregarded until proven by detailed studies. However, in the absence of a plethora of studies regarding MSG, the anecdotal evidence has been used as a springboard to inspire studies as well as other actions by organizations such as the Food and Drug Administration.

The FDA, which is responsible for most food labeling, is scrutinizing the additive and other food ingredients that include it. Although MSG is currently classified by the FDA as Generally Recognized as Safe (GRAS), many people at the FDA have made statements that point to its still-evolving status. The FDA declares some additives as GRAS. It declares some other additives as GRAS but with the note that further study is needed. Ruth Winter's *A Consumer's Dictionary of Food Additives* lists many additives for which the FDA states, "GRAS status continues while tests are being completed and evaluated."

The government actually *never* feels confident enough about any additive to give it a fully clean bill of health. A document from the Food Safety and Inspection Service (FSIS) of the U.S. Department of Agriculture (USDA) states "Additives are never given permanent approval. FDA and FSIS continually review the safety of approved additives to determine if approvals should be modified or withdrawn." Of course, you don't receive information that an additive is Generally Recognized as Safe but still judged to need further testing when you see such an additive listed on a product label.

Trade lobby groups like the Glutamate Association of the United States and the International Food Information Council (an association supported by the food and beverage industry) often state that MSG is completely safe and has never been proven otherwise. They point out that MSG is "generally recognized as safe" by the FDA. They state that no matter how many consumers complain, no one has ever been proved truly sensitive to MSG.

But statements from FDA representatives acknowledge that a number of people are sensitive to MSG. "We believe those sensitive to MSG have been advised by their physicians where it is," said Judy Quick, deputy director of the division of Standards and Labeling in the Food Safety and Inspection Service of the FDA, to *The New York Times.*

In another *New York Times* article, L. Robert Lake, director of compliance at the FDA's Center for Food Safety and Applied Nutrition, stated that food labeling is under review and might be revised so that seasonings and natural flavorings that contain MSG will have to be labeled as such on a food's ingredients list.

Seasonings and natural flavorings often contain MSG, but hydrolyzed proteins added to foods always contain it. Although the FDA has not done much to let consumers know of its concern regarding MSG and ingredients containing it, Lake's statements show that the concern is there, even if it's kept mainly behind closed FDA office doors.

"FDA policy requires food makers to state if MSG is added to their products," Lake told *The New York Times*. "It is also our intent that hydrolyzed vegetable proteins should be declared on the label." In direct conflict with that intent, the article went on to say, is a rule on the FDA's books stating that hydrolyzed vegetable proteins can be called a natural flavoring and be labeled as such.

"We are thinking about revising the regulation," Lake said. "Hydrolyzed vegetable protein should be clearly labeled, and if industry is not doing so, they should know better." In an industry in which making changes for health reasons is like pulling teeth— and often is done only in the presence of extreme government or consumer pressure—how manufacturers can be made to "know better" remains to be seen. The FDA sends a confusing message. Its official MSG policy is one thing, but the statements that indicate its concern about the additive are another.

The studies that are still the most relied upon when it comes to MSG were conducted in the early 1970s by John Olney, a neurophysiologist at Washington University School of Medicine in St. Louis. Prior studies had shown that young rodents force-fed high doses of MSG developed brain lesions. The studies led many to believe that the same results might occur in the still-developing brains of children who consume foods containing MSG.

The concern regarding brain damage arose from the fact that glutamate, which is found naturally in large quantities in the brain, acts as a neurotransmitter. This means it stimulates brain cells. If, however, it is released in large quantities—as can happen during a stroke—it actually becomes a toxin and can stimulate brain cells so much that they die.

Olney conducted tests on seven species of infants, including monkeys and rats. He did not force-feed them huge amounts of MSG, but rather simulated the amount comparable to what a young child might get from eating a bowl of canned soup. Olney found MSG-related brain damage that resulted in obesity, growth retardation, and reproductive dysfunction.

You might have a hard time today finding MSG as an ingredient in baby-food products, but that was not the case when Olney first conducted his studies. Although the FDA did not take formal action, after the studies, almost all baby-food manufacturers removed the substance from their foods.

Olney's studies are still so well regarded in the scientific community that doctors at a recent meeting of the Social Issues Committee of the Society for Neuroscience brought them up again and presented them to the FDA. They requested that the FDA look further at the relationship between MSG and brain damage.

Olney is not the only researcher to have determined such a link. A scientific status summary on MSG by the Institute of Food Technologists' Expert Panel on Food Safety and Nutrition, which generally supports food additive use, pointed out that Olney's finding that "MSG can induce brain damage and a variety of other toxic effects in rodents has been confirmed by numerous investigators, including Abraham et al. (1971), Lemkey-Johnston et al. (1974), and Nemeroff et al. (1977)." They also pointed out that one other study conducted resulted in no brain damage.

Asthma may be triggered by the ingestion of MSG. Dr. Moneret-Vautrin from the Clinic for Immunology and Allergy in Nancy, France, wanted to know how MSG might affect asthmatics. He gave thirty asthmatics a dose of 2.5 grams, which is less than half a teaspoon. He considered that a fairly large amount, but one that could easily be found in a standard American or European meal. Moneret-Vautrin's dosage provoked an asthma response in two of the thirty patients. Moneret-Vautrin, as well as Drs. Allen, Baker, and Delohery, also found that there could be a delay of up to twelve hours in the development of MSG-induced asthma. Study results were reported in the *Journal of Allergy and Immunology*.

MSG researcher and author George Schwartz responded to the French finding by writing, "In view of the 10 million asthmatics in America, it would appear at least 750,000 may be triggering their asthma condition with their daily MSG intake. Having worked as an emergency room physician in many hospitals, I can attest to the frequency of asthma as a presenting complaint. Usually the medical team is too busy providing relief to the patient to take a detailed history of the patient's last few meals. Thus the relationship between MSG and these asthmatic crises easily may go unrecognized."

Physicians like Schwartz point out that much of the public is unaware of some of the basic facts about how MSG differs from seasonings commonly added to food. Ordinary seasonings have an effect on the food, but MSG has an effect on the person.

"When you think of a food or compound like salt or pepper or cinnamon that is added to food, the perceiver can say, 'That adds an interesting taste to my food,' " said Schwartz, who has testified before the FDA about MSG. "But MSG, which has been referred to as a 'mouth aphrodisiac,' has no taste; its purpose is to cause an electrical reaction in the mouth to make your taste sensation longer. MSG is a drug which acts directly on the taste buds, altering their sensitivity." Schwartz warns consumers that if they eat foods laced with MSG day after day, their taste buds may eventually become somewhat desensitized.

Even though MSG produced in factories appears chemically identical to glutamate found naturally in foods, Schwartz and others maintain that, as with many other chemically produced food additives, there is a big difference. In fact, Schwartz believes the reaction in many people to MSG might actually be caused by something in the chemical extraction process.

SURPRISING INGREDIENTS IN WHICH MSG LURKS

Let's say you are one of the many people who actively has been avoiding products that contain MSG, or perhaps you would like to begin doing so after reading about the FDA's statements and studies like Olney's. Can you just read the ingredients on a label to find out whether a product contains MSG?

No. As the tuna fish example at the beginning of this chapter demonstrated, that unfortunately is not the case. A product may state "No MSG added" but still contain hydrolyzed vegetable protein or some other hydrolyzed protein as an ingredient. Each dose of these hydrolyzed proteins will automatically include up to 50 percent MSG. In addition, ingredients such as spices, natural flavorings, and vegetable broth are allowed to and often do contain MSG.

As Lake of the FDA stated to *The New York Times*, companies "should know better" than to add MSG-containing substances without mentioning their true ingredients. However, that's just the point. Many of them seem to know better but at the same time attempt to find more ingenious ways to hide that knowledge.

Food Engineering, a trade journal directed toward food manufacturers, gave this advice to its readers:

"In an effort to help food processors develop more seasoned foods while retaining a 'healthy' image, Takeda U.S.A. introduced Amiflex—hydrolyzed vegetable protein. Although this ingredient offers a high concentration of glutamic acid among other amino acids, it can be labeled as 'seasoning.'" The article went on to say that one variety of Amiflex contains just under 40 percent sodium glutamate.

On their own, hydrolyzed proteins generally have an MSG content of 12 to 20 percent. Some food manufacturers, however, add MSG to the hydrolyzed protein. If that is done, the MSG content can surge to 40 or 50 percent. There is no way for you to know which kind of hydrolyzed protein is used in a given food.

Currently, there is no way to tell whether a product—say a frozen dinner—that says it contains spices, natural flavorings, or other ambiguous ingredients actually contains MSG. You could call the consumer service line advertised on many product labels; but you may find, as Schwartz did, that the consumer service representatives often do not know if those ingredients contain MSG. The best sources at a food company are the food technologists actually involved in making the foods. But they're usually unavailable to the general public.

Here is a partial list of the food ingredients in which MSG may lurk.

Always Contain MSG:

Hydrolyzed proteins.	Sodium caseinate.
Autolyzed yeast.	Calcium caseinate.

May Contain MSG:

Spices.

Seasonings.

Natural flavorings.

Flavorings.

Vegetable broth.

Broth.

Malt flavoring.

High-flavored yeast.

Yeast extract.

Soybean extract.

Textured soy protein.

It may seem difficult, but you can avoid MSG. Don't consume products that contain straight MSG—or any of the ingredients listed above—and you'll be well on your way to an MSG-free diet. And, by cutting down on the kinds of processed foods that tend to contain such additives, you'll be doing yourself a dietary favor in other ways as well.

21

What Is Organic?

"I could buy stickers that say 'organic' and put them on all my produce, even though it wouldn't be true, and so can anybody else," said Vito Scattaglia, who owns Farmer's Mart, a large farmer's marketplace that has operated in Littlerock, California, for more than forty years.

Scattaglia goes to the Los Angeles produce mart three times a week and often sees prominent health food stores in attendance. "In their stores it says it's 'organic,' " he said. "But I know they get a lot of that from the produce mart just like me."

Indeed, even if vendors are not purposely mismarking their produce as organic, many are unwittingly selling produce that is labeled organic when it really is not.

Thomas Harding, a Pennsylvania organic farmer who is founder and past president of the Association for Organic Agriculture, recently asked retailers gathered at the National Nutritional Foods Convention in Las Vegas how they know the batches of produce they get from suppliers are really organic. Many health food stores and mainstream markets, Harding said, may get one batch of apples or other produce from one supplier and another batch from a second and then sell them mixed together at the store, all under the banner of "organic."

Harding and Scattaglia were pointing out two of the pits—as in pitfalls—that are often at the heart of fruits and vegetables labeled "organic." To many consumers, "organic" has become a buzzword associated with "healthful" that leads them to toss produce with such a label into their shopping carts without any further questions.

Organic foods—a multibillion-dollar business—can be better for your health, but it is essential to understand exactly what organic really means to food and why there is a movement gaining steam nationwide to standardize laws and criteria involved in certifying food as organic. Many of us care about this issue. A recent Louis Harris poll of 1,250 people, for example, showed that more than 30 percent had changed their eating habits because of concern about pesticide chemicals in foods.

HOW IS ORGANIC DEFINED?

"From a scientific perspective, all food from vegetable and animal sources is 'organic' because food is derived from a living organism and contains carbon in the chemical structure. Therefore, it is more accurate to refer to 'organically produced' or 'organically grown' foods on the basis of method of husbandry than on the basis of some criterion of the final product," wrote researchers in *Organically Grown Foods: A Scientific Status Summary by the Institute of Food Technologists' Expert Panel on Food Safety and Nutrition.*

The food technologists then go on to point out why trying to get the low-down on "organically grown" produce can often be difficult. "A federal definition for organically grown food does not exist," they wrote, "nor are there any federal standards for production of organic foods or regulation and supervision for the use of the term on food labels. A number of states and regional growers' associations have developed definitions for organically grown food, and some have established certification programs and guidelines for organic growers. However, the definitions, certification programs, and guidelines, some of which include lists of materials allowed for and/or excluded from use, vary from state to state."

Eighteen states have passed laws or regulations defining "organic" for labeling purposes. Fewer than a dozen of those states have hired staff or financed inspection programs to certify that organic farmers meet certain standards.

Different states define "organic" in different ways. Oregon

passed a law prohibiting the use of certain fertilizers for two years and certain pesticides for three years before a harvest can be called organic. The law in California, however, has only a one-year waiting period. In states where there are no laws, you could be buying produce labeled organic from a farmer who just a few months before soaked his soil with pesticides.

WHY DO PEOPLE WANT TO BUY ORGANIC FOOD?

Although it may be difficult to find foods that are truly organically grown when there isn't even a standardized definition of organic foods, there are awfully good reasons many of us want to eat such food. In fact, another Louis Harris Organic Index poll showed that 84 percent of Americans would prefer organically grown fruits and vegetables. About 65 percent cited the long-term health benefits as the most important reason for eating organic produce.

And with the torrent of pesticides and chemicals that are used on American crops, many experts think the public's desire to switch to organic—even without standardized regulations—is a step in the right direction. Harding, for example, states that when he was boy in 1940 there were only 200,000 pounds of pesticides being used per year in the United States. Today, almost 3 billion pounds are being used. Approximately 400 of the 600 registered pesticide ingredients currently in use were, according to the journal *Earth News*, approved before the EPA was assigned the task of regulating them. The EPA admitted to *Earth News* that many of those 400 ingredients would not be allowed on the market if they were up for approval today.

Some ingredients in pesticides have been shown to contribute to the causing of cancer. Fans of pesticide use argue that this has often been corroborated only with people who, like farm workers, have had extensive contact with pesticides in the fields. But the health-concerned don't want even slight residues of such deadly chemicals on the foods they eat. I don't. Do you?

The scary thing is that official comment on this issue, like much of the official comment regarding issues of food safety, is ambiguous. Even though the comment may make it sound like our food is *probably* safe, the wording makes it clear that there are no guarantees. Take a look, for instance, at this part of "Pesticide Research," a scientific status summary report from an expert panel of food technologists concerning organic foods (all emphases are mine):

"The National Research Council recently reported that hypothetical dietary oncogenic [cancer] risk *appears* to be concentrated in a relatively small number of pesticides and crops. Nearly 80 percent of the *estimated* oncogenic risk from all 178 food uses of the 28 compounds that constituted the committee's risk assessment was *estimated* to result from residues of 10 pesticides on only 15 different foods. . . . [Researchers] Doll and Peto [in a separate study] concluded that pesticide contamination of food *seems* unimportant as a factor in cancer mortality. Furthermore, the U.S. Office of Technology Assessment concluded that *most* cases of cancer are not caused by carcinogenic exposures in the food supply, water, pharmaceuticals, work environment, air, water, or soil. Instead, *according to the best interpretation of the evidence currently available,* most cases result from lifestyle factors such as smoking or exposure to sunlight."

The preceding summary report was geared to food technologists, possibly to make them feel somewhat secure about the use and development of questionable pesticides. But how can such interpretations be of comfort to the cancer victims who are *not* part of the majority that does not develop cancer because of pesticides? I'm sure they don't care that *apparently most* cancer patients didn't get cancer the same way they did. And, if the government boasts that "nearly 80 percent of the estimated dietary cancer risk from the 178 food uses of the 28 compounds that constituted the committee's risk assessment was estimated to result from residues of 10 pesticides on only 15 different foods," then why, since the number is so small, wouldn't they develop a different—a safe— pesticide or other growing means to replace those ten pesticides?!

"PESTICIDE RESIDUE-FREE": ANOTHER BUZZWORD IN OUR MARKETS

Before we look at ways to ensure you are actually buying organically grown foods, and at the best steps to cleanse your produce if it isn't organic, let's take a look at a related craze sweeping through many of our supermarkets. The trend is to call produce "pesticide residue-free." This claim cashes in on our tremendous interest in buying safer produce, and it needn't involve organic foods.

Some markets on the West Coast, for example, have been advertising some of their fruits and vegetables as "produce laboratory tested Nutri-Clean; certified; contains no pesticide residues!" Certification businesses like Nutri-Clean have popped up nationwide. Organic farming experts, however, have expressed a number of points of concern.

Let me start the ball rolling with one reminder: Remember, these are businesses. Market Data, a research firm, has reported that the United States organic foods industry, at retail prices, is valued at about $2 billion. By 1995, it is estimated the industry will be about a $4-billion one. The growth has been astounding. The industry was valued at just $174 million in 1980, $893 million in 1988, and $1.25 billion in 1989. My point is that some businesses are being created simply to take a bite out of this huge and wildly growing market.

There are lots of other points to consider as well. "Analytical testing of fruits and vegetables [for pesticide residue] can sometimes be a big deception," said Harding. "There are many factors that are not taken into consideration when testing for residue. So there's no 'detected' residue—that doesn't mean the pesticide hasn't infiltrated the fruit or vegetable itself. It could be inside."

Some experts are concerned that many consumers who see "pesticide residue-free" labels in stores will believe the terminology is interchangeable with the word "organic."

Ideally, "the definition of organic means that no synthetic pesticides can be used in the first place. Testing for pesticide residue means that pesticides may very well have been used but weren't detectable by the time the produce hit the store's shelves," said Mark Lipson, executive secretary of California Certified Organic Farmers, a Santa Cruz-based statewide group of volunteer organic farmers whose primary function is to check that growers who are certified by the state are following correct procedures.

"Also, with pesticide residue testing, you're primarily testing for specific pesticides. If you don't know exactly what's been used, it can't be tested for. Some tests, too, are prohibitively expensive and therefore not conducted," said Lipson, who has been an organic farmer since 1984.

HOW DO I FIND ORGANIC FOODS?

In light of the facts presented in the previous section, you may want to treat produce labeled "pesticide residue-free" as though it had no such label. When you are walking down the aisles of your favorite supermarket or health food store, how, then, can you know which produce is truly organic? The trouble is you can't know for sure, even when it's labeled "organic." Experts suggest the best tactic is to look for products that are not only labeled organic but clearly state they have been "certified" organic and give the name of the organization that has certified them. You should also not be shy about asking your grocer or produce department manager exactly from where and whom produce labeled "organic" is purchased. Then you could consult an or- ganics organization to find out if the suppliers are reputable growers.

A list of reputable organizations that certify organic food through- out the country may be obtained by writing to: Americans for Safe Food, 1501 16th Street N.W., Washington, D.C. 20036. Another good source of information is Mothers and Others for Pesticide Limits, c/o Natural Resources Defense Council, 1350 New York Avenue N.W., Washington, D.C. 20005. For $2.50, they send you a fifty-page con- sumer report. Plus, the California Certified Organic Farmers offers a free list of outlets that sell California-certified organic produce. Write to them at P.O. Box 8136, Santa Cruz, California 95061.

WHAT TO DO IF YOU CAN'T BUY ORGANIC

Many of us will not be able to find organic produce in our markets. However, regular produce looks fine to the naked eye, so is there really any reason for concern? Often, there is no pesticide residue on the produce available to us. However, studies do show reason for concern. An FDA study, for example, revealed that pesticides were detected on more than half the spinach, lettuce, and domestic greens in the United States, as well as on more than half the samples of imported fruits. Apples are sprayed with more pesticides per acre than any other major United States crop. Routine FDA tests show that about one of every two apples contains residues.

What can be done? You may want to peel fruits and vegetables before eating them. However, that gets rid of some of the important fiber. Washing fruits and vegetables is another alternative, but remember that in light of the billions of pounds of pesticides now in use, our produce needs more than a quick rinse using water alone. Invest in a scrub brush for use exclusively on your fruits and vegetables. And, although the EPA is not banning all pesticides that have been shown to be harmful, they do have a suggestion about what we should do when questionable produce reaches our home. When he was chief of the EPA's Dietary Exposure Branch, Charles Trichilo often recommended that consumers should wash produce with a brush as well as a small amount of dish soap that contains no artificial colors or perfumes. Produce may also be soaked in ample water to cover it, with a few drops of dish soap added. Rinse and scrub carefully to remove any soapy residue.

When produce is waxed—as in the case of many cucumbers, apples, bell peppers, eggplants, peaches, and tomatoes—special care should be taken. Waxes can't be washed away but can seal in pesticide residues. If you suspect produce is waxed, you may want to peel it before consuming it.

Here are some specific suggestions from the Center for Science in the Public Interest:

- Eat as usual: Bananas, corn, grapefruit, oranges, melon, and other peeled fruit. When grating orange or lemon peel for cooking, use organic produce or wash thoroughly.

- Wash thoroughly: Cabbage (discard outer leaves), cauliflower, celery (trim leaves and top), cherries, grapes, green beans, lettuce, potatoes, and strawberries.

- Peel if waxed: Cucumbers, eggplant, tomatoes (blanch first for easy peeling), and peppers (roast first for easy peeling).

- Peel: Carrots.

- Buy organic, if possible: Apples, broccoli, peaches, pears, and spinach.

22

Vegetarian and Macrobiotic Diets

Gail Chandler became a weight-loss guru without even trying. It wasn't writing a book or appearing on television that brought dieters to her door. It was the aroma of her homemade vegetarian lunches.

Chandler, finance manager at a recreational vehicle dealership in Lancaster, California, had eager recruits appearing at her desk when she was munching on vegetarian lunches to help maintain her forty-pound weight loss. One day, a male coworker stopped by and told her that her lunches always looked and smelled so good. Would she, he asked, bring him lunch every day, too? He offered to pay her fifty dollars a month to do it.

"Just from eating the lunches—he didn't alter his other meals— that guy lost thirteen pounds in one month," said Chandler, who has since opened a catering company and begun teaching vegetarian cooking. "Soon, I was making lunch every day for a dozen people who had heard about the results."

Until about six months before Chandler started making lunches for those dozen people, she had battled a lifelong weight problem. Each partial stride she made to vegetarianism prompted about a fifteen-pound, almost immediate, weight loss. However, this last time, she switched for good to a diet that avoids all meat, poultry, fish, dairy, and other animal products. Without counting calories, within two months she dropped the extra forty pounds from her five-foot, seven-inch frame.

Chandler is one of a growing breed of vegetarians—those who turn to the lifestyle specifically to improve their health and/or lose weight. Like Chandler, these converts to vegetarian diets may become as steadfast in their commitment to eat no animal products as those who chose vegetarianism for humane reasons. More and more, in fact, the standard diets prescribed by mainstream dietitians and government agencies mirror vegetarian and macrobiotic diets (which we'll describe later in this chapter). That is because mainstream sources of nutrition information have begun recommending more vegetables and whole grains and less protein, especially red meat.

In fact, you may already be a "semi-" or "part-time" vegetarian. If you routinely avoid meat and select poultry and fish and start each morning with whole-grain cereal, then many health agencies, such as the Mayo Clinic and the American Dietetic Association, already refer to you as "semi-vegetarian." Let's take a look further down that vegetarian path on which so many of us are taking those first few preliminary steps. After that, we'll take a quick look at macrobiotics, a structured vegetarian way of eating.

HEALTH BENEFITS OF VEGETARIAN DIETS

You don't have to commit completely to a vegetarian eating plan to see the tremendous health benefits. Like Chandler and others, you might want to begin by tilting your dietary choices in a slightly vegetarian direction and then deciding whether to take it further. Just a slight shift is the case with diets that are often advised for people trying to avoid cancer.

"Because of their low-fat, high-fiber content, [vegetarian diets] have numerous health benefits," writes the Mayo Clinic in its *Nutrition Letter* as words of encouragement. "Even if you don't see yourself giving up meat or other animal proteins entirely, eating more plant-based foods can help you reduce total fat, saturated fat, and cholesterol in your diet." That's, of course, due to the fact that only animal products contain cholesterol—although a few vegetable products, like palm and coconut oil, do contain saturated fat, which can lead your body to produce cholesterol.

"The main reason people choose a vegetarian diet is the increasing evidence of its healthful effects," continues the Mayo Clinic.

The American Dietetic Association couldn't agree more. In "Position of the American Dietetic Association on Vegetarian Diets," a technical support paper in *ADA Reports*, they write, "Vegetarians are at lower risk for non-insulin-dependent diabetes and have lower rates of hypertension, osteoporosis, kidney stones, and gallstones than non-vegetarians. Mortality from coronary artery disease is lower in vegetarians than non-vegetarians. Vegetarians have lower rates of mortality from colon cancer than does the general population. That may be due to dietary differences which include increased fiber intake, decreased intake of total fat, cholesterol, and increased intakes of fruits and vegetables."

TYPES OF VEGETARIAN DIETS

Although many health-conscious people are switching to plant-based diets, vegetarianism and macrobiotics are no dietary newcomers. Vegetarianism dates back to ancient India, the Far East, and ancient Rome and Greece. Vegetarian diets are classified according to the types of animal foods that are excluded:

- *Vegans.* Vegans are total vegetarians. They exclude all animal sources of food. This includes meat, poultry, eggs, fish, milk, and all other dairy products.

- *Lacto vegetarians.* This group will consume milk and other dairy products but excludes meat, eggs, fish, and poultry.

- *Lacto-ovo vegetarians.* In addition to dairy products, this group will eat eggs. However, lacto-ovo vegetarians do not eat meat, fish, or poultry.

- *Semi- or part-time vegetarians.* This is considered the fastest-growing group of vegetarians. Some might avoid red meat but still consume poultry and fish. Others avoid all saturated animal fats.

CAN YOU GET ENOUGH NUTRIENTS
ON A VEGETARIAN DIET?

Although the test results are in and vegetarians as a group have
less disease and weigh less than non-vegetarians, some vegetarians worry that by excluding meat they may not be getting
enough amino acids (the building blocks of protein) or other
nutrients. However, vegetarians who eat eggs, milk, or cheese
generally do not need to worry about amino acid or other
nutrient deficiencies because their diets include animal protein.
Stricter vegetarians may need more careful meal planning. And
a vegetarian who never eats any animal products will need to
get vitamin B_{12} from other sources. Strict vegetarians also must
ensure they are consuming enough vitamin D, iron, and calcium. The Mayo Clinic recommends the following sources to
make the vegetarian's task easier:

- For calcium: Soybeans and other legumes, tofu, broccoli, mus-
  tard, collard and turnip greens, spinach, bok choy, okra, almonds, sesame seeds.

- For iron: Legumes (some examples: dried beans, peas, lentils,
  chickpeas), tofu, green leafy vegetables, whole wheat, dried
  fruit (some examples: apricots, peaches, raisins). Absorption of
  iron is enhanced by vitamin C. Good sources of vitamin C are
  citrus fruits and juices, tomatoes, broccoli, strawberries, peppers, dark green leafy vegetables, and potatoes with their skins.

- For vitamin B_{12}: B_{12}-fortified soy milk, B_{12}-supplemented meat
  analogues (substitutes, usually from soybeans, made to resem-
  ble meats such as hot dogs, ground beef, sausage, and bacon),
  B_{12}-tablets (also called cobalamin supplements), B_{12}-fortified
  whole-grain cereals.

- For Vitamin D: Vitamin D-fortified margarine, vitamin D supplements. Also, sunshine activates a chemical in your skin and
  converts it to vitamin D. But with the current skin cancer scare,
  which has kept many people out of the sun, it is possible for
  some people to get too little sunlight. The following, for example, describes a woman who happens to have been a vegetarian
  since she was a teenager. (It comes from an article I wrote for

syndication on the subject.) Can any of you busy, successful, yet sun-starved readers relate to her?

"Lois Blane, a young attorney from Tarzana, California, opens a door in her condominium's living room, walks down some stairs to her indoor garage, hops into her red sports car, and speeds off to her skyscraper *L.A. Law*-like corporate law office in downtown Los Angeles. After a long day racking up her billable hours, she hops back into her car, which is parked under the building, rushes home, whips out her electric garage door opener, and is back in her three-level condo—often without ever having been touched by a single ray of sunlight."

In Chapter 18, I recommended taking supplements—the least being a multitvitamin and mineral tablet that includes 100 percent of the RDAs for most vitamins, calcium, and iron and even more of such especially important vitamins as A, C, and E. This would, of course, be especially recommended for vegetarians.

WHAT IS MACROBIOTICS?

The macrobiotic diet is Japanese in origin. It is based on the Oriental theory that health is created by balancing the yin and yang, which are the universal forces of expansion and contraction. Through diet, the body's energy is harnessed to work with yin and yang.

A macrobiotic diet is free of most animal foods. The traditional macrobiotic meal consists of about 50 percent whole grains (usually brown rice), about 30 percent cooked vegetables, 10 percent soup (usually a miso—fermented soybean paste—broth), and 10 percent beans and sea vegetables. Seasonal fruits and nuts and seeds are also sometimes used. And those people living in temperate climates may eat moderate amounts of white-meat fish and certain shellfish. Like many vegetarian diets, macrobiotic diets are exceptionally low in fat.

MAKING THE TRANSITION TO A MACROBIOTIC DIET

Since a macrobiotic diet is a vegetarian diet, all the great health benefits of vegetarianism also apply. Many people are making the transition to a macrobiotic diet for just such health reasons.

But can eating a diet that relies on sea vegetables and fermented soy paste be tasty? You bet. To see if you might be interested in eating the macrobiotic way, take a look at Table 21.1, a shopping list of macrobiotic foods and ingredients. (It comes from the excellent book *Making the Transition to a Macrobiotic Diet* by Carolyn Heidenry.)

Table 21.1 Macrobiotics Menu

Vegetables

Acorn Squash	Leeks
Bok Choy	Lettuce
Broccoli	Lotus Root
Brussels Sprouts	Mushrooms
Burdock	Mustard Greens
Buttercup Squash	Onions
Butternut Squash	Parsley
Cabbage	Parsnips
Carrot Tops	Peas
Carrots	Pumpkin
Cauliflower	Radishes
Celery	Red Cabbage
Chinese Cabbage	Rutabaga
Collard Greens	Scallions
Crookneck Squash	Sprouts
Cucumber	String Beans
Daikon	Swiss Chard
Endive	Turnip Greens
Hubbard Squash	Turnips
Kale	Watercress

Whole Grains

Barley	Oats
Brown Rice	Rye
Buckwheat	Sweet Rice
Corn (whole)	Wheat
Millet	

Beans and Bean Products

Aduki Beans
Black Soy Beans
Black Turtle Beans
Chick Peas (Garbanzo)
Great Northern Beans
Kidney Beans
Lentils

Navy Beans
Pinto Beans
Red Lentils
Tofu
Tempeh
Soy Beans
Split Peas

Sweeteners

Apple Butter
Barley Malt
Currants
Dried Apples
Dried Apricots

Dried Peaches
Dried Pears
Maple Syrup
Raisins
Rice Syrup

Grain Products

Bread (whole grain flour)
Bulghur
Cornmeal
Couscous
Cracked Wheat
Flour (whole grain)
Mochi

Noodles and Pasta
  (whole grain)
Oatmeal
Rolled Wheat, Rye, or Barley
  Flakes
Steel-Cut Oats

Sea Greens

Agar Agar
Arame
Dulse
Hiziki
Irish Moss

Kelp
Kombu
Laver
Nori
Wakame

Fruits

Apples   Peaches
Apricots   Pears
Blueberries   Plums
Cantaloupe   Raspberries
Cherries   Strawberries
Chestnuts   Watermelon
Grapes

Specialty Items

Kuzu   Shitake Mushrooms

Seasonings

Corn Oil   Sesame Oil
Ginger Root   Tamari Soy Sauce
Mirin   Umeboshi Plums
Miso   Umeboshi Vinegar
Sea Salt   Vinegar (Brown Rice)

Snacks

Cookies   Peanut Butter
Corn Chips   Popcorn
Crackers   Rice Cakes
Granola   Sesame Butter
Muesli   Tahini
Muffins

Beverages

Amasake   Herb Tea
Barley Tea   Kukicha Tea
100% Fruit Juice   Spring Water
Grain Coffee

Seeds and Nuts

Almonds	Sesame Seeds
Peanuts	Sunflower Seeds
Pecans	Walnuts
Pumpkin Seeds	

Vegetarianism and macrobiotics are terms that can intimidate some people, who think that commitment to such ways of eating is an all-or-nothing proposition. However, as the research I've reported shows, even small steps in the direction of a vegetable- and grain-based diet can yield great health rewards.

23

Alcohol

It took John Oake of Cleveland five years to admit he was an alcoholic, three years before he was sober, and two more years before he even had his first sips of what he thought was "non-alcoholic" beer. However, those few sips could have cost him his hard-won sobriety. Like Oake, many consumers, whether they are recovering alcoholics or just part of the wave of drinkers who are looking for non-alcoholic alternatives, probably don't realize that the "non-alcoholic" brew they pride themselves on drinking actually may contain some alcohol—possibly enough, researchers say, to shove a recovering alcoholic like Oake off the sobriety wagon.

Like food labeling (discussed in Chapter 17), alcohol labeling can harbor some real surprises. Whether it is a type of wine that has more alcohol than the hardest of liquors but is packaged to look like low-alcohol wine coolers and marketed toward women and teenagers (groups with a typically lower weight and who therefore may become intoxicated more quickly), or whether it is "non-alcoholic" brews that really contain alcohol, we consumers should be up on the facts about alcohol.

We also should be aware of the health facts. Virtually every mini-market and corner bar in the country sells alcohol. Unfortunately, not as readily available are the results of the studies that have pointed out the health risks associated with what many people consider even "moderate" consumption of alcohol. Unlike Oake, many people have been sipping a margarita or two weekend after weekend for decades without ever having an alcohol problem or becoming an alcoholic. Do you have an alcohol "problem"? If you are drinking even "moderate" amounts of alcohol without being aware of the health implications or the labeling ploys like those just listed, then you may, in fact, have a problem.

ARE LIQUOR MANUFACTURERS TRYING TO CONFUSE YOU?

Before we take a look at the results of some of the studies regarding alcohol and health, let's scrutinize those "non-alcoholic" beers and other types of alcohol that might be misleading. Certainly, if you are a recovering alcoholic, you probably don't want to be drinking anything with even a little alcohol in it. And if you are among the growing number of people who choose not to drink, you also would not want to drink a "non-alcoholic" beverage that actually contains alcohol. However, that's just what happens when you drink most "non-alcoholic" beverages.

By law, according to the Bureau of Alcohol, Tobacco and Firearms, beverages labeled "non-alchoholic" can contain up to one-half of 1 percent of alcohol. (The average regular-strength beer has 3.5 or 4 percent alcohol.) Is this really enough to trigger a drinking episode in a recovering alcoholic? Some experts have found that to be the case.

Ruben Zepeda, a counselor for Charter Oak Hospital in Los Angeles, saw two of his patients rehospitalized for their alcoholism after suffering a relapse when they started drinking non-alcoholic beers.

"When alcohol goes in the body at whatever level, it incites the neurological system all over again," Zepeda said. "[My patients] had a full relapse. They drank one can, two cans, until they totally deteriorated and had to go back into the hospital."

Dr. Ronald Alkana, a University of Southern California professor of pharmacology and toxicology, also has warned against the consumption of non-alcoholic beverages. "Why take a chance if you're trying not to drink?" he said. "That's dangerous." Dr. Alfonso

Paredes, a UCLA psychiatry professor and the chief of substance abuse programs at the West Los Angeles Veterans Administration, said that drinking non-alcoholic beverages that contain some alcohol is "just like Russian roulette for the alcoholic."

If your intention is not to drink any alcohol, be sure to read the small print on labels carefully.

PACKAGING CAN BE MISLEADING

Are you drinking a wine cooler or a potentially deadly "wine fooler"? At least ten youths in Washington, D.C., were fooled enough by hard alcohol that was packaged like a wine cooler to end up in a hospital emergency room with alcohol poisoning. Certain "fortified" wines—packaged to look like wine coolers and most often sold alongside them—were drunk by the youths and others across the country as though they were wine coolers. However, the fortified wines, which until recently were packaged like hard alcohol, are often 40 proof. That is 20 percent alcohol by volume, compared with the 4 percent of most wines and wine coolers. Drinking one 12-ounce bottle of fortified wine is the equivalent of five shots of 80-proof vodka, said Ray Chavira, who has been a member of the California State Advisory Board on Alcohol-Related Problems and the Los Angeles County Alcohol Policy Coalition.

The issue became so serious that in 1991 U.S. Surgeon General Dr. Antonia Novello held a news conference about the fortified wines. She said that just two 12-ounce bottles of fortified wine drunk in an hour by a 100-pound person could cause death from alcohol poisoning. If a 150-pound person drank that amount, she said, he or she would be legally intoxicated. Many of the companies that have packaged their fortified wines like wine coolers have been feeling pressure from Novello and various groups to change their labels.

In the meantime, this is just another issue that proves it is important, maybe even life-saving, to read even the tiniest print on the labels of the products you buy and to be aware how much alcohol by volume should be in a given type of product—for instance, 4 percent in a wine cooler.

ALCOHOL AND YOUR HEALTH

About two-thirds of all American adults drink alcoholic beverages, but 10 percent of the drinkers (about 7 percent of the total adult population) account for at least half the consumption, according to studies done at the University of California at Berkeley. At least 90 percent of all college students drink. And more than one-quarter of the nation's college students are chronic abusers of alcohol, according to research by Alan Berkowitz and H. Wesley Perkins of Hobart and William Smith Colleges in Geneva, New York.

If you do drink alcohol, I'm certainly not here to tell you to stop. But as with anything concerning nutrition or health, it is essential to understand what alcohol—a drug—does inside our bodies. Some people think of alcohol the way they think of caffeine—as simply an ingredient in beverages they enjoy. However, caffeine and alcohol are most definitely drugs. Even moderate consumption of alcohol can have effects on almost every body organ, especially the liver, brain, and nervous system.

So what happens when alcohol enters your body? From the instant it enters, it can alter the body's functioning. It is quickly absorbed by the walls of the gut into the blood stream, where it is transported throughout the body. Excessive amounts of alcohol can then disrupt nerve cells, block the flow of nutrients, destroy liver cells, and damage heart muscles. Also, alcohol possibly disrupts normal immune responses. This was reported, among other places, in *You Are What You Drink*, studies publicized by Joseph Barbato, a director for the Alcoholism Council of Greater New York.

The body can metabolize only about one-quarter ounce of alcohol an hour. Amounts greater than that start to accumulate in the blood stream and affect the brain and other organs. In the brain, alcohol acts as a narcotic. Like a sleeping pill, it can put to sleep certain nerve cells that affect behavior.

It doesn't take an excessive amount of alcohol to trigger serious changes in your body. Alcohol, according to the Mayo Clinic, increases the frequency of heart muscle contractions, which can lead to heart palpitations or a fluttering feeling in the chest. If you have coronary heart disease, then alcohol, combined with exercise, also puts you at risk for heart attack. "If you have narrowed coronary arteries, strenuous levels of exercise may cause chest pain, which can be a warning for heart attack. Drinking alcohol, however, lessens your awareness of this signal," reported the Mayo Clinic.

Alcohol also appears to be associated with the development of high blood pressure. Researchers at Stanford University found that as alcohol intake increased, so did blood pressure. After age fifty, the link between alcohol consumption and hypertension appears strongest, although a connection was shown in all study subjects age twenty and older.

It has long been thought that alcohol can affect how the skin looks. Studies in Finland have now shown that alcohol consumption can lead to the development of psoriasis, an incurable skin disorder that produces red scaly patches that may itch, crack, and bleed. Researchers at the National Public Health Institute in Helsinki asked about 150 men with psoriasis about their alcohol consumption during the year before they developed the condition. The men had drunk, on average, the equivalent of four glasses of wine a day, compared with about two daily glasses for 280 men questioned about other, less serious skin disorders. The psoriasis sufferers also reported that once they had contracted psoriasis, alcohol consumption caused the condition to flare up.

Psoriasis and heart problems can affect anyone who consumes alcohol; everyone who drinks is at risk. But there are specific groups of individuals with their own special risks, and the health community discourages them from drinking any alcohol at all: Pregnant women (studies have shown possible fetal birth defects); breast-feeding mothers (what you eat and drink, your baby eats and drinks); people on medication (alcohol can cause deadly combinations with certain medications); and diabetics (since alcohol can interfere with blood sugar metabolism, a physician should be consulted before a diabetic starts to drink alcohol).

IS ALCOHOL CAUSING YOU WEIGHT GAIN OR DEPLETING YOU OF VITAMINS?

Like refined sugar, alcohol is the epitome of the term "empty calories"—those that offer no nutrients. Yet, although you are ingesting absolutely no nutrients, you are getting plenty of calories. (For a listing of some common alcoholic beverages and the amount of calories they contain, see Table 23.1.)

Table 23.1 Calorie Content of Alcoholic Beverages

Beverage	Size of Serving	Calories
Beer		
	12-ounce can	140–164*
	light, 12-ounce can	96–134*
Gin/rum/vodka/whiskey		
	80 proof, 1 fluid ounce (small jigger)	65
	90 proof, 1 fluid ounce (small jigger)	74
	100 proof, 1 fluid ounce (small jigger)	83
Wine, white, alcohol 11.5% by volume		
	3½ fluid ounces (small wine glass)	80
Wine, red, alcohol 11.5% by volume		
	3½ fluid ounces (small wine glass)	76
Wine cooler		
	12-ounce bottle	150–200**
	light, 12-ounce bottle	135**

*The calorie content of beer varies depending on the brand. All light beer must be labeled to show the calorie content, but regular beer labels do not have to show calorie content.

**The calorie content of wine coolers varies depending on the alcohol content (which generally ranges from 4 to 7 percent alcohol by volume) and the amount of sweeteners (such as fructose, dextrose, high-fructose corn syrup) that a particular brand contains. Only the "light" wine cooler labels must show calorie content.

Source: *Mayo Clinic Nutrition Letter.*

You were probably aware that the alcohol you drink contains calories (although perhaps not as few as you'd thought), but did you ever stop to consider that your beer, wine, or martini might also be chock-full of additives? As they are in foods, additives are used in many alcoholic beverages. However, alcohol is overseen by the Bureau of Alcohol, Tobacco and Firearms, not by the FDA, which oversees food labeling. Therefore, different rules apply.

For example, many ingredients and additives do not even have to be listed on alcohol packaging, because they are considered "trade secrets." All in all, almost sixty additives are legally allowed in beer alone without label declaration, according to the bureau. Some of the common "secret" additives in liquor include sodium bisulfite, petroleum, ether or chloroform solvents, and artificial foam stabilizers.

In addition to ingesting additives unwittingly when you consume alcohol, you might be causing vitamin depletion within your body. Much of alcohol advertising is now aimed at fitness-minded, active people. Many of those people may be part of the crowd who made vitamin supplementation a multibillion-dollar business. But how many of us realize that as we gulp alcohol we may be negating attempts we've made through diet and supplementation to ensure that we are getting enough vitamins and minerals?

Alcohol keeps your body from utilizing folic acid, a B vitamin needed by the bone marrow to produce red blood cells. Drinking alcohol can also lead to iron and zinc deficiencies, which are related to long-term immunity problems and, in the short term, less immunity from colds and flus. Vitamins A, B, and C and the mineral magnesium can also be partially depleted by the consumption of alcohol.

HASN'T ALCOHOL CONSUMPTION BEEN SHOWN TO BE GOOD FOR ME?

No studies have ever shown hard alcohol in any amount to be good for us. However, recent well-publicized studies have shown that small amounts of wine may have some protective qualities. Does this counteract all the negative changes even moderate amounts of alcohol can cause in your body? Most experts don't think so.

The protective effect most linked to small amounts of alcohol involves a possible reduction of heart disease. Medical researchers in France showed that the higher consumption in France of red wine may have something to do with the lower incidence of heart disease in their country. However, these results (unlike results of tests proving how destructive alcohol can be) were anything but firm. This is how the researchers described their findings in a health journal: "When 16 healthy men each consumed three or four glasses of red wine every day for about two weeks, several positive changes occurred in the blood which, if maintained over a period of time, *might* [emphasis mine] reduce their risk of having a heart attack."

However, such information can be confusing to the average drinker. For example, it had earlier been shown that all wine drinking—white wine included—could help prevent heart disease. It was later shown, though, that white wine increases cholesterol, which can increase heart disease risk. Therefore, it is no longer recommended as a protector. Since the researchers are not sure what it is about red wine that may help protect against heart disease, it could get taken off the protector list someday, too!

AM I REALLY DRINKING THAT MUCH?

It doesn't take a lot of alcohol to cause serious health problems. Although it takes a certain amount of drinks to be considered legally intoxicated (.10 percent blood alcohol in many states), your health can often be affected by amounts much smaller than that.

For example, a chart from the government's Department of Public Safety indicates the amount of alcohol necessary for people of different weights to reach the .10-percent blood alcohol level. For a 100-pound person, the number of six-ounce glasses of wine that would have to be drunk within one hour is three; for a 160-pound person, the number of glasses is five; and for a 200-pound person, the number of glasses is six.

However, the government's health officials are a bit more stringent about what they consider "heavy drinking." The Centers for Disease Control (CDC), for example, considers heavy drinking to be an average daily consumption of one ounce or more of ethanol (the chemical name for alcohol). That translates into about two beers, cocktails, or glasses of wine. That is the amount the CDC took into consideration when compiling its statistics on "heavy drinkers." Heavy drinkers, they reported, run a seven times greater risk of liver cirrhosis than non-heavy drinkers. At least 46 percent of the cirrhosis deaths among United States men, and at least 15 percent of cirrhosis deaths among the nation's women, are attributable to heavy drinking, according to the CDC. More than 25,000 people died of chronic liver disease in 1990, according to the CDC, and almost half of those deaths were associated with alcohol.

Alcohol-related deaths, of course, involve more than just liver disease. They include household and highway accidents caused by intoxication, plus many other tragedies. Alcohol-related mortality ranks as the fourth-leading cause of death in the United States, behind heart disease, cancer, and strokes. And, according to government statistics, alcohol isn't just taking its toll on the elderly after years of cumulative use. Rather, based on current life expectancies, the average number of years of potential life lost per alcohol-related death was thirty-one!

People who are trying to consume a healthier diet need to think about what they are drinking as well as what they are eating. As you lift your glass of wine, beer, or whiskey, you should be aware of exactly what is in it and what it does inside your body once you sip it. Many health-concerned people have made mineral water or fruit juice their beverage of choice. Armed with the facts, you may want to do the same.

24

The Food Pyramid

After years of promoting the "four basic food groups," which many nutritionists and researchers argued were outdated and based on old research, the government did away with the groups in May 1992 and instead decided to teach everyone how to climb their new food pyramid.

Actually, there were seven basic food groups mentioned in 1946, when the United States Department of Agriculture (USDA) first let the public know what they thought would be the best food choices. Those groups were: Leafy green and yellow vegetables; citrus fruit, tomatoes, and raw cabbage; potatoes and other vegetables and fruits; milk, cheese, and ice cream; meat, poultry, fish, eggs, dried peas, and beans; bread, flour, and cereals; and butter and fortified margarine.

A few years later, the USDA streamlined the seven groups into four: Fruits and vegetables; breads and cereals; meat, poultry, fish, and eggs; and dairy products.

Many nutrition organizations criticized the basic four campaign. They said there was too much emphasis put on the meat/poultry and dairy groups, which tend to harbor many high-fat, high-cholesterol foods. There was not much distinction made by the USDA between how many servings from each group an individual should have. The government has listened and is now recommending a complex-carbohydrate, low-fat, high-fiber diet.

The food pyramid makes it clear that grains and cereals and fruits and vegetables are the champs when it comes to nutritious food choices. The least desirable food groups are placed in the small upper end of the pyramid; the more desirable groups are in its huge base, forming the foundation. (See Figure 24.1.)

What follows is a description of each level of the pyramid based on the USDA's recommendation. In parentheses after each description is a slight adjustment I've made based on the recommendations of those who promote the most natural, "whole food," disease-prevention type of diet.

Fats, oils, and sweets form the tiny peak of the pyramid. The USDA's recommendation is to use fats and sweets sparingly. (Whenever possible, do not use saturated fats. Use monounsaturated and polyunsaturated fats. For a complete discussion of fats and oils, see Chapter 13. When it comes to sweets, avoid refined sugar and high-fructose corn syrup, which is chemically manufactured. Eat foods sweetened with honey; with fructose, which is unadulterated fruit sugar; and with other unrefined sweeteners. For a complete discussion of sweeteners, see Chapter 12).

The next level on the USDA's pyramid is shared by the milk, yogurt, and cheese group—recommendation: two to three servings—and the meat, poultry, fish, dry beans, eggs, and nuts group—recommendation: two to three servings. (Many nutrition organizations recommend that eggs, because of their cholesterol count, be eaten only two or three times a week. Red meat should also be consumed only, at most, a few times a week. Stick with skinless poultry, and fish that is low in cholesterol. White-meat poultry has less fat than dark meat. Shellfish like shrimp and lobster have significant amounts of cholesterol. As far as dairy products, cheese, and yogurt go, choose non-fat and low-fat varieties. Also, a number of brands of regular and frozen yogurt are both non-fat and sweetened with fruit or fruit juice rather than refined sugar.)

The next level, moving toward the bottom of the USDA's pyramid, is occupied by vegetables—recommendation: three to five servings—and fruits—recommendation: two to four servings. (Eat your fruits and vegetables fresh and raw whenever possible. When cooking vegetables, steam them rather than boil them. And, most importantly, take the higher serving suggestion. That is, for

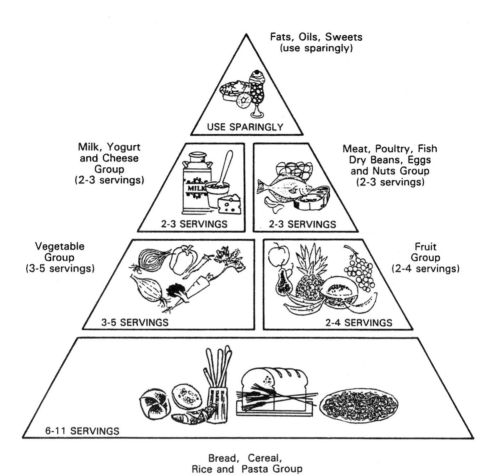

Fats, Oils, Sweets
(use sparingly)

USE SPARINGLY

Milk, Yogurt
and Cheese
Group
(2-3 servings)

Meat, Poultry, Fish
Dry Beans, Eggs
and Nuts Group
(2-3 servings)

2-3 SERVINGS   2-3 SERVINGS

Vegetable
Group
(3-5 servings)

Fruit
Group
(2-4 servings)

3-5 SERVINGS   2-4 SERVINGS

6-11 SERVINGS

Bread, Cereal,
Rice and Pasta Group
(6-11 servings)

Figure 24.1. Current USDA Food Guide Pyramid.

cancer prevention, try to eat nine servings of fruits and vegetables
a day, concentrating on leafy green and red or orange vegetables.)

The base of the pyramid, its whole foundation, is occupied by
the bread, cereal, rice, and pasta group. The USDA recommends
six to eleven servings from this group daily. (Use whole-grain,
non-enriched, non-fortified, high-fiber breads and cereals without
any sugar, additives, or chemicals. Use non-enriched brown rice.
"Quick" brown rice is a new product on supermarket shelves. For

pastas, use a non-enriched whole-wheat flour or a substitute flour such as artichoke flour.)

Scaling the new food pyramid isn't difficult. But remember that it, like the old RDAs, represents the minimum level of nutrients needed. Follow the "optimal" suggestions added above and not only will you make it to the top of the pyramid, you'll probably feel like you're on top of the world!

Conclusion

The statistics are scary, aren't they? Millions upon millions of people are affected by the ravaging diseases brought on in large part by a poor diet.

Heart disease. Cancer. Stroke. They are the three leading killers in this country. All, as I've shown throughout this book and as reflected in our country's medical literature, have strong links to diet and are mainly preventable diseases.

All those deaths and disabilities are the negative side hidden behind the counter of the virtual smorgasbord of eating choices we have. Step out in front of that counter and survey the vast lineup of tasty food that visionary health researchers have displayed for you. Making the right choices day after day can quite possibly help you prevent cancer and heart disease and even live to an age much closer to that most scientists believe we were meant to reach—about 125.

IMMUNITY AND LONGEVITY

Dr. Estella Ramey isn't trying to squeeze out an extra 44 years just for her own pleasure. Rather, the 76-year-old Maryland-based endocrinologist is an expert on aging, metabolism, enzymes, and hormones, and she thinks it entirely reasonable that people should expect to live to be 120 years old. Many other researchers agree with her.

In fact, Ramey was giving a low-number estimate when she described the 120-year life span (if proper nutrition is followed) to a gathering of the American Association of Oral and Maxillo-facial Surgeons. Actually, Ramey said the human heart, if it receives a normal supply of blood and good nutrition, has a life expectancy of 150 years and the brain 200 years.

No matter what your expected life span, we are already wasting many years, according to scientists. Since 1982, the Centers for Disease Control has published the number of years of potential life lost from common causes of mortality. In 1990, for example, assuming a paltry 65 years as the normal life span, Americans suffered a loss of more than 12 million years of potential life to all causes. This included losses to nutrition-related diseases, such as 1.8 million years to cancer, another 1.5 million years to heart disease, and 250,000 years to stroke.

As glum as the thought of all those lost years is, when healthful eating is employed, it seems the results are diametrically opposite. Recent studies at both the National Institute on Aging's Gerontology Research Center in Baltimore and the University of New Mexico of nearly 2,000 healthy men and women over age 65 showed that people who consistently eat a healthful diet add an average of 8 years to their expected life spans.

These new studies, as well as past ones, link beta-carotene (which the body uses to make vitamin A) and vitamins C and E to the increased life span. These vitamins are becoming known as powerful anti-oxidants, meaning they can help neutralize destructive cells. "These nutrients may well be the secret ingredients that help stymie development of major diseases and could slow down the aging process of cells," said Dr. Richard Cutler of the National Institute on Aging.

If eating right can help build immunity, then it can help people live longer. As this book has shown, eating certain foods can, in fact, help reduce the risk of cancer and heart disease and even make the body fight the onset of cancer.

Other studies also tie eating well to increased immunity. A first-of-its-kind recent study showed that eating a low-fat diet boosts immunity in humans. Cutting the amount of fat in the diet is associated with a rise in the activity of natural disease-killing cells, reported researchers at the American Health Foundation in New York. These immune cells are credited with hunting down and knocking out cells infected with viruses, as well as cancerous cells.

Other research has linked as simple an act as eating breakfast—the most important meal of the day—every day with increased life span. And, as you age, do you need to worry about every gained pound? Actually, it looks as though it is healthier to gain a moderate amount of weight as you age than not to gain any weight. More than ten years of research by Dr. Reubin Andres and colleagues at the Gerontology Research Center at the National Institute on Aging recently confirmed some findings from the long-term Framingham (Massachusetts) Heart Study and the Harvard University Alumni Study. Those studies showed that people who gain a moderate amount of weight steadily throughout their adult lives have lower mortality rates than people who gain no weight at all or people who gain a large amount of weight. However, other studies have shown that, as you age, even though it is healthful to gain a bit of weight gradually, you should still be cutting your caloric input because your metabolism slows down. Cutting caloric input has been linked to longevity.

A FOOD PLAN FOR YOUTHFULNESS AND LONGEVITY?

Although the average life span for a human being is currently 74 years, most experts agree that number could get quite a bit higher. Dr. Roy L. Walford, a UCLA pathology professor considered one of the country's top authorities on aging, thinks that number may reach 125 years or more.

"[The dietary research] is based on many years of animal experimentation in my own laboratory at the UCLA Medical School and in other laboratories in other major universities in the United States," Walford wrote in his book *The 120-Year Diet*. "There is no doubt at all that the life span of animals can be extended by more than 50 percent by dietary means, corresponding to humans living to be 150 or 160 years old."

The trick, most experts say, is adjusting your calories so you are always eating a low-calorie yet nutrient-packed diet. Reducing calories in such a manner has been shown to extend animal life in the experiments of Walford and many others.

"Since rejuvenation means limiting calories, it also means getting the maximum number of vitamins, minerals, proteins, carbohydrates, fiber, and essential fatty acids per calorie from our diet. Those foods highest on the nutrient density scale are the best fuel for our bodies," said Dr. Gershon Lesser, an author and researcher.

WORST FOODS

A lot of regulars have chosen the Doughnut Inn in Palmdale, California, as their breakfast haunt, and their favorite meal choice is a twin cinnamon doughnut or a cinnamon nut cluster doughnut, according to manager Tim Chor. Nationally-acclaimed nutrition advisors Earl Mindell and Jane Brody, however, say they think those regulars would be better off with just a dash of cinnamon thrown over their shoulders for nutritional luck.

Throughout many states, crowds pour in every day to Bob's Big Boy restaurants for their breakfast bars. The all-you-can-eat bonanzas include everything from eggs to apple pancakes and a lot of bacon. More than one hundred slices of bacon go into a tub, and the tubs are replaced many times over during the run of the breakfast bar, according to a representative of the restaurant chain. At each restaurant is one cook whose only job is to keep cooking bacon. Mindell and Brody would rather the cook were chopping fruit and that the crowds, as long as they laid off the heavy dressings and cream soups, would make their way instead to Bob's soup-and-salad lunch bar.

And they say that those across the country who drop in at A.M./P.M. Mini Markets to fill up on their perennial two-hot-dogs-for-eighty-eight-cents special might be better off restricting their filling up to gasoline, a gallon of which not too long ago also was going for eighty-eight cents.

Hot dogs, bacon, and doughnuts are among the foods that appear on the lists of the all-time worst foods of some of the country's top nutritionists. Too often, experts stress, the health-conscious will jump into a very restrictive diet that mandates only a few foods be eaten. It might be better, Mindell and Brody say, to make a list of the ten worst foods and simply avoid them.

"Most of these foods, and you'd better put the word food loosely in quotation marks, are trash foods—that's what the British call them. And, in fact, most of these foods are pure junk," said Mindell, R.Ph., Ph.D., and author of the best sellers *Earl Mindell's Vitamin Bible* and *Unsafe at Any Meal*.

The foods on Mindell's list of those to avoid at all costs are bacon, diet and regular soft drinks, doughnuts, fried foods, hot dogs, mayonnaise, packaged snack cakes, powdered drink mixes, shakes, sugared cereals, and white bread.

The list distributed by Brody, author of the best-selling *Jane Brody's Nutrition Book*, seconds the motions against bacon, doughnuts, fried foods, soda, and sugared cereal.

As far as doughnuts go, Brody writes in her advisory, they are "worse than no breakfast at all. Not only do doughnuts have the sugar and white flour that we should be cutting back on, but they're fried. Doughnuts put your blood sugar out of whack, and they don't stay with you. By the end of the morning, you'll be in bad shape." Mindell said he agrees that it would be better to have no breakfast at all than to eat a doughnut.

Brody cautions against grabbing most brands of granola bars instead of a doughnut. Granola bars, perhaps surprising some aficionados, ended up on her list of the ten worst foods.

"Whoever said they are healthful? Granola is a high-fat, high-sugar cereal," she warned. "I use it only as a garnish. Granola bars are simply high-calorie cookies. The latest version—the granola candy bars—are no better for you than a Milky Way."

Mindell suggests in *Unsafe at Any Meal* baking homemade granola without using sugar. (See recipe on page 204.)

Bacon is a culprit because of its high fat content—some bacon gets as much as 95 percent of its calories from fat—and its high levels of nitrites, which may cause cancer.

"Anything, just to be considered bacon, must have nitrites," Mindell said. "It is also high in salt and sugar. If someone's eating a lot of bacon, I'd suggest making sure they supplement with vitamins E and C and beta-carotene—which may be cancer protectors."

Nitrosamines, which form in the body after you eat nitrites, are carcinogens. Cured meats like bacon add nitrites to the diet and nitrosamines to the body.

Homemade Granola

2 tablespoons honey
2 tablespoons sunflower (or sesame seed) oil
⅛ teaspoon vanilla
1½ cups oats
¼ cup wheat germ
½ cup chopped peanuts
½ cup chopped almonds
½ cup sesame seeds
½ cup pumpkin seeds
½ cup sunflower seeds
½ cup raisins

Mix together the honey, sunflower (or sesame seed) oil, and vanilla, and pour over a mixture of all the other ingredients. Spread the mixture on a shallow, flat pan, and bake at 325°F for 10 minutes, stirring to prevent sticking. Continue baking for another 10 minutes, or until the granola is toasty brown.

Source: *Unsafe at Any Meal* by Earl Mindell, R.Ph., Ph.D. New York: Warner Books, 1987.

Mindell offers some tips if you don't want to quit bacon cold turkey. Bacon grease, which contains nearly four times as many nitrosamines as bacon, should not be used for cooking, he advises. Microwaved bacon is better because fewer nitrosamines are produced, although the fat content remains the same. And don't inhale the aroma of bacon while it is cooking any more than is absolutely necessary, because some nitrosamines are vaporized during cooking and are easily inhaled.

White bread made the worst-foods list because it lacks fiber, and since its formula is standardized by the government, it can contain more than one hundred food and chemical additives that do not need to be listed on the label.

BEST FOODS

After sounding off about what they consider the worst foods, what do these and other nutrition experts consider to be among the top foods when it comes to good nutrition? Well, you'll find plenty of those listed throughout this book, and following are a few of Brody's and Mindell's favorites.

Brody's list includes broccoli, Brussels sprouts, cabbage, carrots, cauliflower, fresh fruits, lentils, oats, pasta, popcorn, potatoes (not fried or chips), skim milk, whole-grain breads, and yogurt.

There is a lot of agreement on Mindell's part. He, too, recommends broccoli, Brussels sprouts, and yogurt. In addition, he is a fan of salmon, mackerel, sardines, and tuna.

Dr. Arnold Fox, a cardiologist and former medical professor at the University of California at Irvine and author of *Immune for Life*, experimented with foods and put together a list of the most nutrient-dense foods available. Other longevity experts have expressed much agreement with Fox's list. Recommended for anti-aging diets, the foods should be used as much as possible—steamed, tossed in salads, prepared in soups, etc. Fox's foods include beans, beet greens, black Chinese mushrooms, broccoli, Brussels sprouts, cabbage, cantaloupes, carrots, cauliflower, garlic, ginger, lentils, oat bran, onions, parsley, peaches, peas, red peppers, scallions, spinach, sweet potatoes, water, and whole grains.

You've probably noticed that many of the foods thought to ensure longevity are the same ones that have been proven to protect against cancer and heart disease and help you lose weight. They are also among the foods you should be eating if you want to eat a natural foods diet rather than an artificial-additive-packed one.

Bibliography

Many sources—health journals, reports of nutrition studies, interviews, and articles—were used as research for this book. References to them are noted in the text. In addition to those sources, the following books were helpful to the author and provide lively suggested further reading for those interested in preventive nutrition and health.

Bennett, William I., M.D., Goldfinger, Stephen G., and Johnson, Timothy G., M.D. *Your Good Health: How to Stay Well, and What to Do When You're Not From Harvard Medical School*. Cambridge, MA: Harvard University Press, 1987.

Crook, William G., M.D. *Dr. Crook Discusses Hypoglycemia*. Jackson, TN: Professional Books, 1984.

Dufty, William. *Sugar Blues*. New York: Warner Books, 1975.

Editors of *Prevention Magazine*, ed. *Complete Book of Vitamins*. Emmaus, PA: Rodale Press, 1984.

Fox, Arnold, M.D. and Fox, Barry. *Immune for Life: Live Longer and Better by Strengthening Your Doctor Within*. Rocklin, CA: Prima Publishing and Communication, 1989.

Garland, Cedric, M.D., and Garland, Frank, M.D. *The Calcium Connection*. New York: G.P. Putnam's Sons, 1988.

Gershoff, Stanley, Ph.D. *The Tufts University Guide to Total Nutrition*. New York: Harper & Row, 1990.

Goulart, Frances Sheridan. *Nutritional Self-Defense: Protecting Yourself—How to Use Nutrition to Counteract the Effects of Your Eight Worst Habits*. New York: Dodd, Mead & Company, 1984.

Heidenry, Carolyn. *Making the Transition to a Macrobiotic Diet*. Garden City Park, NY: Avery Publishing Group, 1984, 1987.

Jacobson, Michael F., Ph.D. *The Complete Eater's Digest and Nutrition Scoreboard*. New York: Anchor Press/Doubleday, 1985.

Lieberman, Shari, and Bruning, Nancy. *The Real Vitamin and Mineral Book*. Garden City Park, NY: Avery Publishing Group, 1990.

Lindsay, Anne. *The American Cancer Society Cookbook: A Menu for Good Health*. New York: Hearst Books, 1988.

Messinger, Lisa. *Turn Your Supermarket Into a Health Food Store: The Brand Name Guide to Shopping for a Better Diet*. New York: Pharos/Scripps Howard Books, 1991.

Neile, Caren. *Banish Allergies Forever*. Boca Raton, FL: Globe Communications, 1991.

Rosenberg, Irene, M.D. *Fat in Your Pocket: Fat Facts Fast*. Hewlett, NY: Wellness International, 1988.

Ross, Harvey M., M.D. and Roth, June. *The Mood Control Diet*. New York: Prentice Hall Press, 1990.

Rowan, Robert L., M.D. *How to Control High Blood Pressure Without Drugs*. New York: Ivy Books, 1986.

Schwartz, George R., M.D. *In Bad Taste: The MSG Syndrome, the Essential Update*. Santa Fe, NM: Health Press, 1990.

Stewart, Clifford, Ph.D. *Cancer: Prevention, Detection, Causes, Treatment*. Wallingford, PA: Hampton Court Press, 1988.

Walford, Roy L., M.D. *The 120-Year Diet*. New York: Simon and Schuster, 1986.

Winston, Mary, Ed.D., and Eshleman, Ruthe. *American Heart Association Cookbook*. New York: Times Books/Random House, 1991.

Index